Re

The Potent Pause

Victor Shamas, Ph.D.
& Jhan Kold, M.S.

Foreword by Dr. Gary Schwartz

REPOSE

The Potent Pause by Victor Shamas, Ph.D. and Jhan Kold, M.S.

Copyright © 2015 by Victor Shamas and Jhan Kold

All rights reserved. No part of this book may be reproduced or transmitted in any form or by any means, electronic or mechanical, including photocopying, recording or by any information storage and retrieval system, without permission from the authors.

Cover Photo by Aryen Hart, featuring co-authors Jhan Kold and Dr. Victor Shamas in Repose.

Dedicated to our shared vision of a world in Repose

Want more joy? Read *Repose: The Potent Pause*. As a healing aid, Repose is better than aspirin. This book should be required reading for every health care provider!

—Amy Weintraub, author of *Yoga for Depression* and *Yoga Skills for Therapists,* founder of the LifeForce Yoga Healing Institute

"Life is lived in the pauses, not the events," wrote Hugh Prather. This powerful teaching quickly comes to life in Repose, which guides us into a simple and accessible experience of the sweet peaceful undercurrent of life. Repose is a grand gift, a revolutionary technique that at once effectively promotes our physical, psychological and spiritual well-being.

—Rubin Naiman, PhD, author of *Hush: A Book of Bedtime Contemplations* and founder of Circadian Health Associates

The practice of pausing to reflect and regroup is a lost art in our culture today. Repose offers an engaging creative way to restore the essential balance point in our hearts and minds, and so in our lives.

—Lisa Thiel, singer-songwriter and recording artist, whose albums include *Circle of the Seasons*, *Songs of Healing*, and *Invocation of the Graces*

The power of the human body for self-healing and transformation is much greater than we realize. Once in a while, something comes along that harnesses this power in new and profound ways. Repose is one of those breakthroughs in the evolution of wellness. Because of its purity and simplicity, Repose will appeal to a large population of individuals seeking balance and wholeness in their lives.

> —Tryshe Dhevney, best-selling Sounds True recording artist and author of *SOUNDShifting: Your Personal Guide to Self-Healing with Sound*

The energy of this book feels amazing. Repose is elegant simplicity, allowing anyone to do it and gain immediate benefits. Repose is a gift that provides healing at a Soul level, naturally allowing you to escape the trappings of the mind, without the complication of how to do it the right way. Repose gives you the opportunity to slow down from the complexities of life, move back to center, and remember who you really are, in only seven minutes. A total win for our busy lives. Thank you for sharing this gift to humanity!

> —Ellie Drew, author of *Way of the Lotus Flower* and founder of the Institute for Conscious Change

Contents

Foreword..8

Introduction...10

Life in Repose..11

CHAPTER 1: What is Repose?..12

Life in Repose: Cara, 24, recent college graduate and lifelong "student of the Universe"..14

CHAPTER 2: Where did Repose come from?................................16

Life in Repose: Karin, 54, teacher and "Swedish Viking Goddess"..........21

CHAPTER 3: How was Repose discovered?..................................23

Life in Repose: Dane, 28, social worker managing programs for at-risk youth...24

CHAPTER 4: Is it meditation?...26

Life in Repose: Renate, 72, grandmother and widow of six years..........27

CHAPTER 5: Is it relaxation?..29

Life in Repose: Monyka, 45, mother, teacher, and creative artist............30

CHAPTER 6: What happens in Repose?..32

Life in Repose: Tom, 61, community leader interested in yoga, health, ecology, and sustainable economies..34

CHAPTER 7: Receptivity and Repose..36

Life in Repose: Martha, 67, acupuncturist and Reiki Master..................40

CHAPTER 8: Which thoughts are most conducive to Repose?...............42

Life in Repose: KC, 72, recovery support specialist..................44

CHAPTER 9: Why is Repose such a "potent pause"?..............46

CHAPTER 10: Where's the proof?..54

CHAPTER 11: Where do we go from here?.............................61

Life in Repose: Victor, age 55, psychologist, author, musician.................63

CHAPTER 12: Adaptations and modifications........................65

Life in Repose: Jhan, age 55, rehabilitation specialist, yoga teacher, and Earth steward..69

Notes..71

Foreword

Do not underestimate the ideas you are about to discover. Repose may seem little more than lying supine with outstretched arms and legs, but the potential ramifications of this simple act may be far-reaching. Based on the significant benefits experienced by those who have tried it thus far, including some of the people whose stories you will read, Repose could have widespread application as a fundamental aid to physical and mental health. Even more exciting than the anticipated impact of Repose are the unexpected consequences.

When the Yale Psychophysiology Center, under my direction, began its program of research on biofeedback in the late 1970's, none of us associated with the center knew that our work would help revolutionize the way society thinks about health and illness, give rise to two new fields of research (behavioral medicine and health psychology), and challenge existing assumptions about human consciousness. Much like Repose, biofeedback started out as an interesting little technique with potential health implications. It turned out to be much more than that.

One of the powerful lessons of biofeedback is that human beings can regulate autonomic functions like heart rate and blood pressure through their conscious intention. The use of the word *autonomic* to identify these functions is driven by the assumption that they have autonomy, operating outside the control of the conscious mind. This assumption turns out to be wrong. Through biofeedback training, individuals can learn to regulate various kinds of processes in their bodies, sometimes in remarkable ways.

Biofeedback training and Repose have something in common. In both processes, the individual receives feedback from the body. The type of feedback may differ. In biofeedback training, this information comes in the form of an external electronic signal indicating autonomic activity, such as the beeping of a heart rate monitor. In Repose, the individual receives internal feedback in the form of physical sensations experienced while lying in an open, receptive posture.

What really sets the two apart is the way the feedback gets used. In biofeedback training, the mind utilizes the signal to control the autonomic activity being monitored. For instance, the person using a heart rate monitor might learn to slow down his or her pulse, which may have certain health benefits such as alleviating stress. In Repose, however, the mind seems to use the feedback from the body to give up control altogether. The authors of this e-book maintain that the physical receptivity of Repose leads to a type of mental receptivity that can have a profound impact not just on health but on consciousness.

For millennia, humanity has sought ways to alter, transform and expand consciousness. Virtually every culture has developed some form of meditation practice with that purpose in mind. Spiritual aspirants may devote decades to mastering such practices. It seems that Repose may induce experiences similar to meditation in a much more effortless manner. Nobody disputes the value of spiritual discipline, but for the majority of people who lack the time or energy to master meditation, Repose may offer a powerful alternative without the learning curve. The accessibility of Repose makes it noteworthy. Because of its combination of simplicity and efficacy, Repose could be appealing to millions of people, which means that its potential impact could be felt globally. That is an exciting possibility, indeed.

Introduction

Imagine a resource that can enhance health, eliminate stress, slow down aging, elevate mood, reduce pain, improve sleep, and increase productivity. Even a single exposure to this resource can energize you and fill you with a sensation of blissful relaxation that lasts for hours or days. Repeated exposure can transform your life in the most positive ways imaginable. When many people share this resource at one time, the effects are magnified exponentially.

This resource does not come in the form of a pill, capsule, cream, or salve. There is nothing to buy. You do not need to attend a costly workshop, watch a training video, or hire a personal coach. It is perfectly portable. You can use it virtually anywhere. The benefits of this resource are so profound, and the cost in terms of time and money so negligible, that the decision to incorporate it into your daily life is self-evident.

The resource is called Repose. This e-book will answer all your questions about Repose and get you started on a path that will enhance virtually every aspect of your life. We will describe the science behind Repose, including research data showing its enormous benefits. You will read about our experiments on Repose and the case studies of people whose lives have been improved by it. Please keep in mind that Repose has only been around a short while. We first discovered it in January 2014. Before a single word was ever written about Repose, thousands of people started incorporating it into their daily routine. This enthusiastic reception is a testament to the profound ways that Repose is transforming people's lives.

Life in Repose

Throughout this book, we will be featuring the extraordinary true stories of individuals whose lives have been changed dramatically by Repose. These stories are told largely in the person's own words, and each feature will include a picture of the person in Repose. You will find a total of 10 "Life in Repose" features, each at the end of a chapter. The last two will tell the unique stories of the two co-authors.

CHAPTER 1

What is Repose?

Repose involves lying on your back on a flat, comfortable surface (floor, bed, carpet, mat, lawn, etc), with arms extended perpendicular to your torso, palms up, legs open, and jaw relaxed, as shown here:

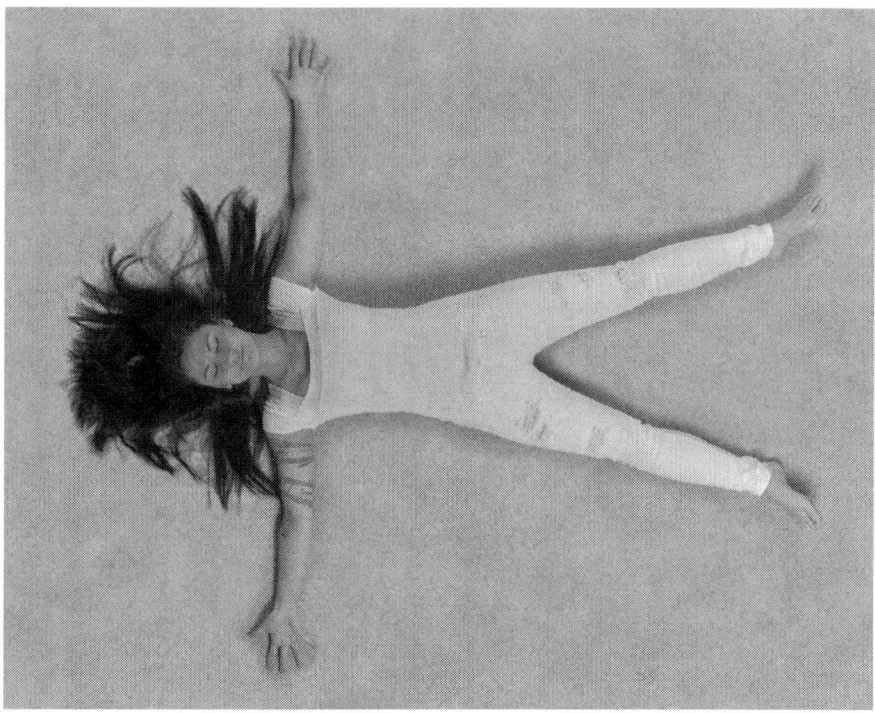

There should be no strain anywhere in the body. When in Repose, arms and legs are never extended beyond their natural comfort level. If possible, Repose should be done in a quiet place, with eyes either open or closed. We recommend doing Repose for seven minutes three times a day at the following times: 9am, 3pm, and 9pm. The idea is to spread the benefits of Repose evenly throughout your day. If you are unable to accommodate these times into your schedule, you may modify the starting times of your three Repose sessions as needed, keeping in mind that Repose is most effective when distributed over the course of your day rather than concentrated in one long session.

Of course, Repose is nothing new. At some point in your life, you may have seen people in this position or tried it yourself. One of the striking things about Repose is that it conveys such a powerful sense of well-being. When we ask people to describe someone lying in Repose, they use the following adjectives: carefree, happy, open, peaceful, receptive, and relaxed. In Repose, all the joints of the body are in an open, extended position: ankles, knees, hips, shoulders, elbows, wrists, and jaw. As we shall see, this openness offers an important clue as to why the benefits of Repose are so profound.

Notice that Repose differs markedly from other supine positions used for relaxation. Some have compared it to the Corpse Pose in yoga, also known by the Sanskrit name *Shavasana*. But in the latter, the arms are extended no more than 45 degrees and the legs are kept relatively close together, which makes a difference in terms of the body's dynamics. Also, Shavasana requires that eyes be closed and awareness be maintained on the breath, whereas Repose does not. In Repose, you can think about or focus on whatever you want. You already know innately how to be in Repose, without needing to be told what to do or think. When in Repose, your body leads and your mind follows. This happens simply, naturally, and without any conscious effort on your part.

Life in Repose
Cara, 24, recent college graduate and lifelong "student of the Universe"

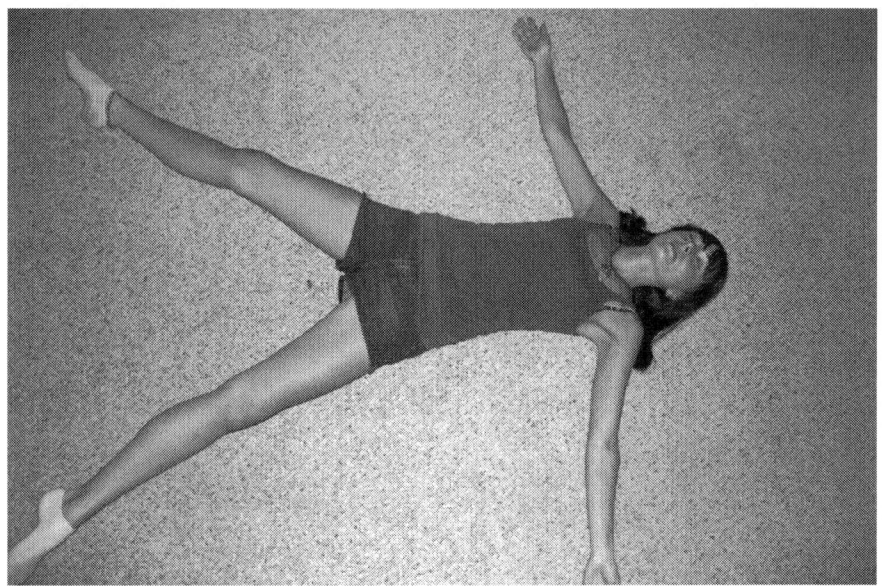

Before learning about Repose, Cara had a meditation practice she did daily while lying on the floor. "Usually, I lie down with my legs almost together and my arms by my side. Once I was introduced to Repose, I started using it as my go-to position instead. Right away, I noticed that it helps me relax faster and I can feel energy moving through me more easily."

Cara tends to use Repose as part of a long, deep meditation she does every morning. "It makes me feel refreshed and focused. When I find I do not have time for my usual meditation in the morning I will just lie in Repose for 5-10 minutes and this short time is enough for me to feel more energized and alert."

Cara began incorporating Repose at a time when she was making a number of lifestyle changes. "I cannot say for sure if Repose was responsible for the many benefits I received during this time, but I do know that my health and well-being have improved greatly since Repose came into my life."

One of the authors of this book introduced Cara to Repose. "At first, my legs were crossed. He suggested that I spread them out wider and extend my arms out more, too. As soon as I was in the correct position I closed my eyes and relaxed. I immediately could feel waves of energy hitting me over and over again like a blanket being fanned over my body. My relaxation deepened as I mentally but loudly thought: *WOW!*"

For Cara, Repose offered an important lesson in surrender. "This is a very open position, and it made me feel vulnerable at first. In our society we are taught to keep our guard up, both physically and mentally. When we assume a closed position, we may be protecting our vital organs but we are also closing ourselves off to all the messages and vibrations that are out there. Lying in Repose feels like I'm letting go of resistance and trusting in the universe. It's a body position that screams, 'I surrender to your will. Send me what I need. I trust you.' I think regular use of this practice could allow people to see that receptivity is not the same as vulnerability. When we open ourselves up like we do in Repose, we find out how powerful it is to simply trust. There is nothing to fear, really, and everything to be gained."

CHAPTER 2

Where did Repose come from?

Repose has always been a part of the human experience, although you might not have been aware of it. If you look carefully, you will find examples of Repose everywhere. Just consider the phenomenon of the snow angel:

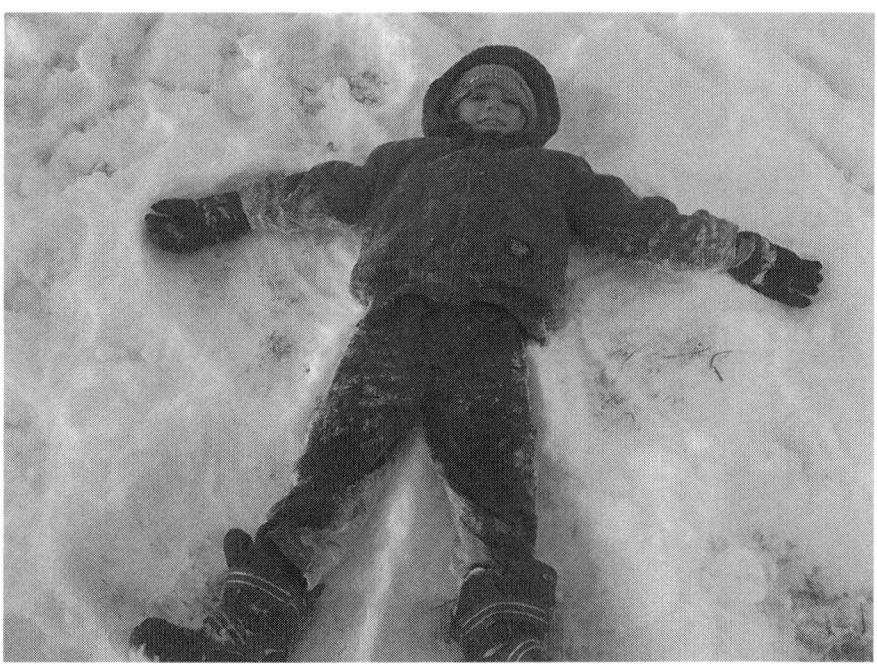

Why is it that so many people feel compelled to lie in the snow in this position? Is the image of a snow angel so beautiful that someone will get cold and wet just to create it? The experience itself must feel so satisfying that people are willing to endure a little cold just so they can have the sensation of being in Repose.

On a beach or sand dune, you are likely to encounter a similar phenomenon, which is that of the sand angel:

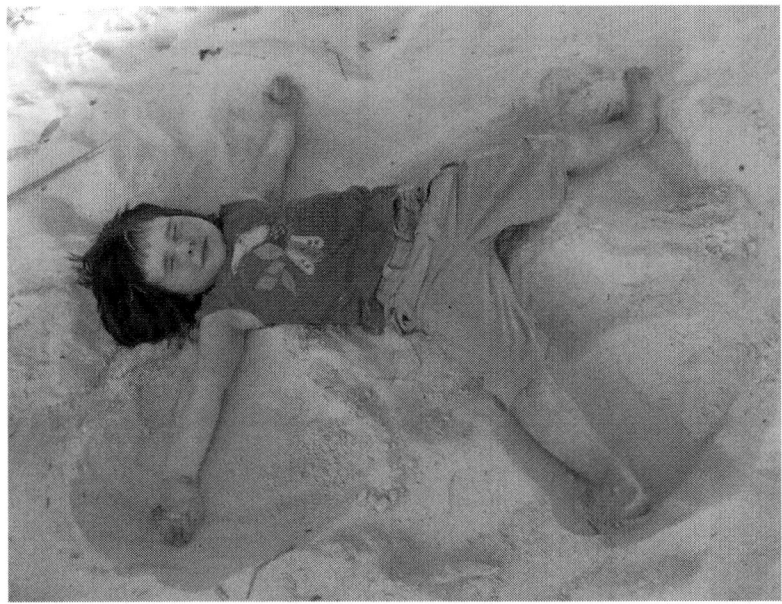

Instead of cold, the creator of a sand angel runs the risk of getting sand into every crack and crevice. But perhaps a major sand removal operation is a small price to pay for a few delicious moments of Repose on the warm, soft sand.

Now, consider the image of a gingerbread man.

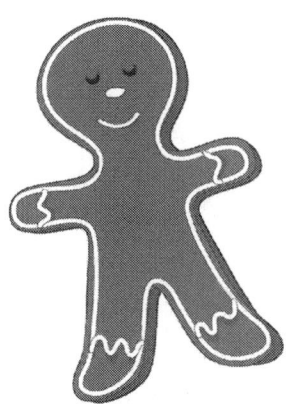

Have you ever noticed that a gingerbread man is always in Repose? One of the reasons that bakers may be drawn to this specific shape is that it conveys good cheer and a carefree demeanor. A gingerbread man provides a vicarious experience of Repose to those who see or consume it.

If you do a Google image search for the word "carefree," you will encounter pictures like this:

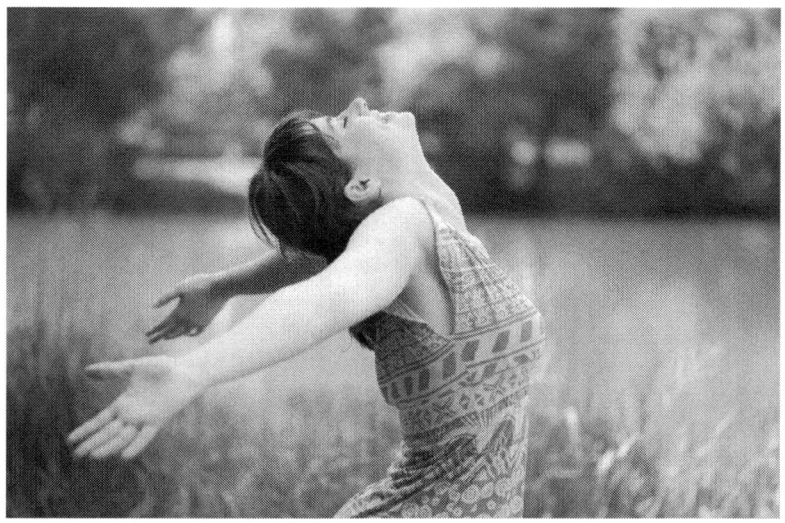

Although the individual is standing instead of lying down, this stance bears a striking resemblance to Repose. Notice the extension of the arms, which conveys the sense of openness and freedom that characterizes someone unburdened by concerns or worries.

We have speculated that part of the reason *Singing in the Rain* is such a beloved film has to do with the prevalence of this carefree stance. Our informal count shows that Gene Kelly and his co-stars assume a standing version of Repose at least 25 times during the course of the movie, most notably in the "Gotta Dance" sequence and, of course, while performing the title song.

Other classic images convey the spirit of Repose. When people are first introduced to Repose, many of them think of Leonardo da Vinci's classic work, known as the "Vitruvian Man." We could never quite understand why Leonardo gave this guy such a stern facial expression, which seems incompatible with Repose, and so we invited artist Aryen Hart to lighten his mood and help him relax a bit. We call this slightly modified version *Repose Man*:

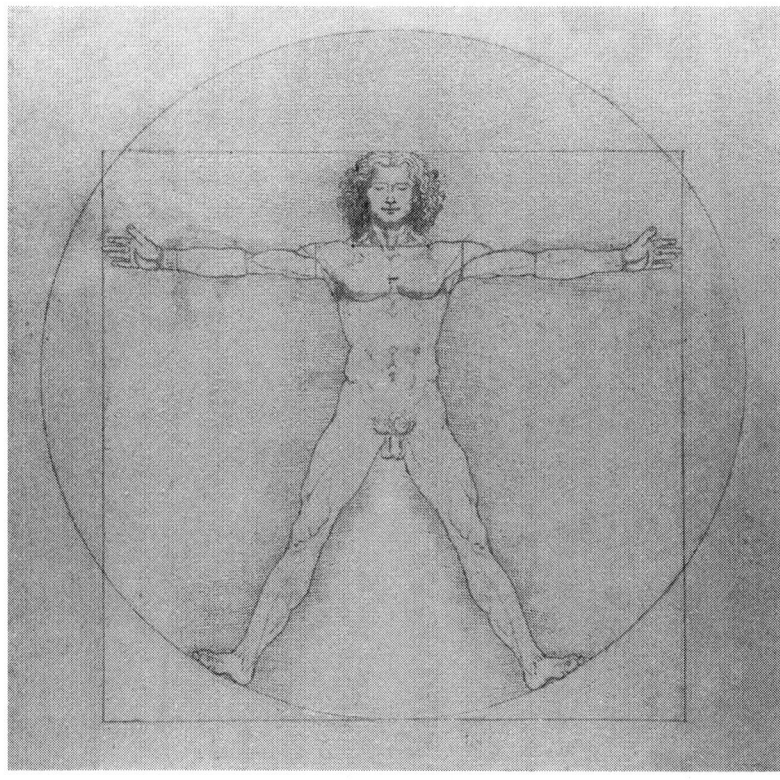

Another standing version of Repose that has captured our imagination can be found on the wall of a small church in Siena. This image depicts Saint Catherine of Siena in rapture. We wonder if Catherine's stance is an expression of her rapture or possibly the cause of it. What if the stance itself serves as a means of inducing rapture? The accounts of individuals who have been doing Repose on a daily basis suggest that this might just be the case.

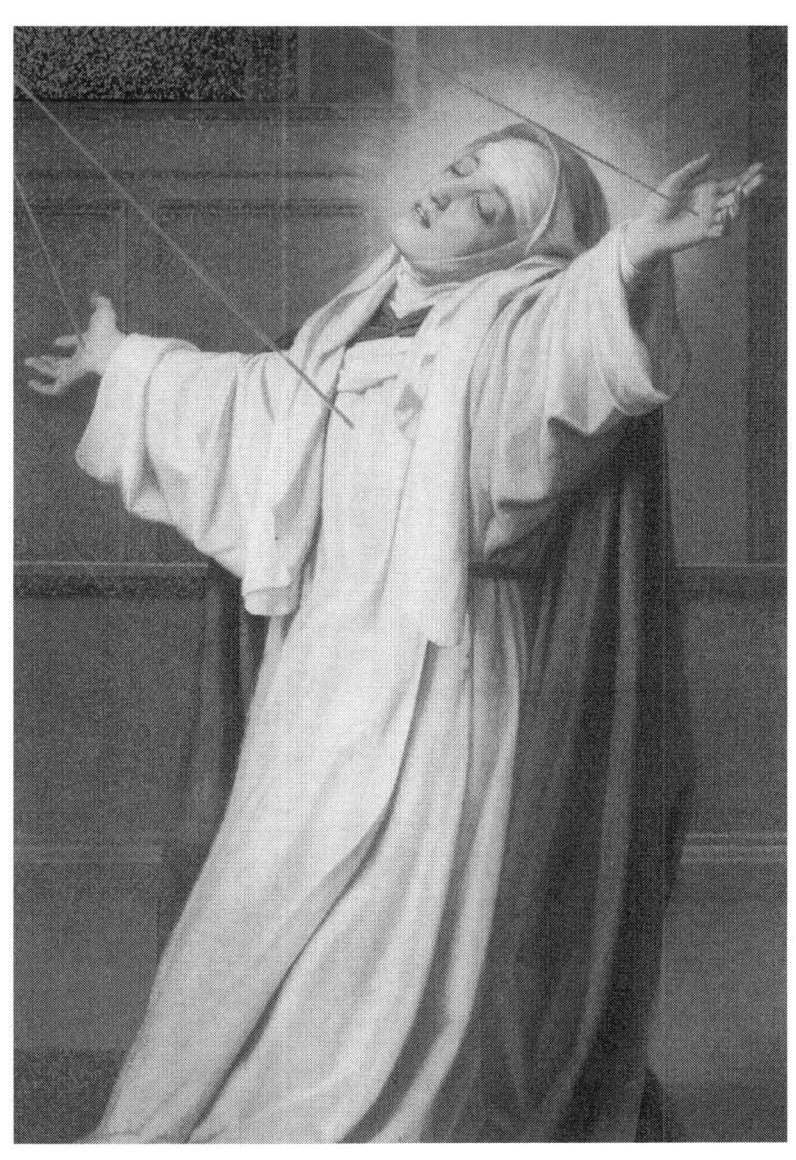

Life in Repose
Karin, 54, teacher and "Swedish Viking Goddess"

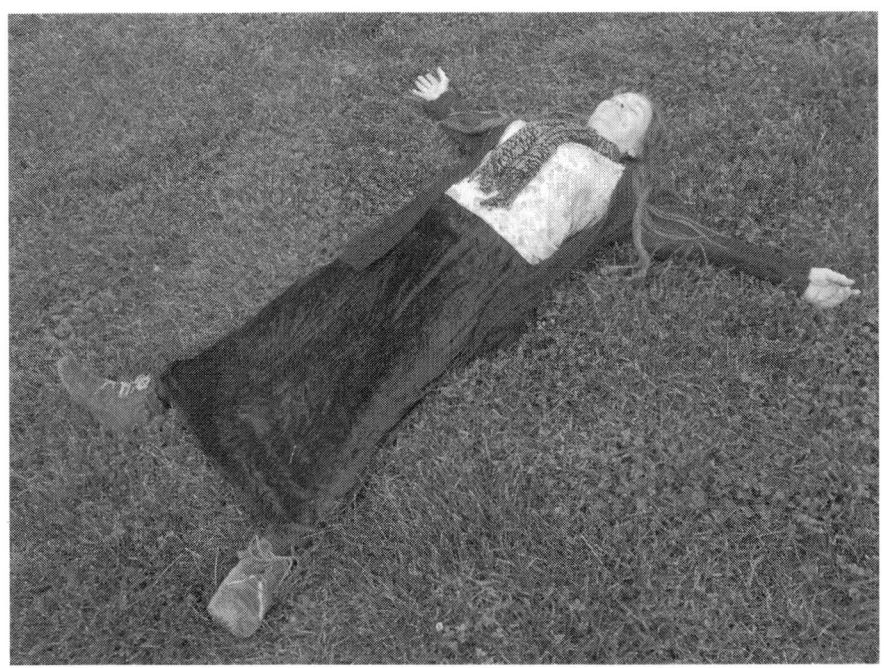

When Repose became part of Karin's daily routine, other teachers would be startled to walk in on her lying on the floor of the staff lounge. Eventually, some of them began joining her. "At first, I noticed subtle changes in attitude among the staff—especially the ones who were taking Repose breaks with me," she remarks. "After a few weeks, the entire mood of our school seemed to shift. It became a much more enjoyable place to work."

Karin continues to start her day with Repose. During her morning Repose session, she uses nature imagery such as beaches, forests or prairies to help her relax and prepare for what lies ahead. "It helps me catch my breath and visualize the kind of day I want to have. While I'm lying in Repose, I focus on the positive and think about ways to manifest it."

For Karin, Repose has been an effective way to deal with traumatic events in her life. "This practice has been such a blessing at a time when I have experienced multiple losses and have had to deal with a lot of sorrow, grief, and stress. It calms me and reminds me of things for which I am grateful."

She has found that Repose can pull her out of negativity and stress pretty quickly. "I just allow my mind to follow my body into a peaceful state, and that seems to stimulate pleasant memories or even humor." Repose has been so effective for Karin that she has even brought it into the classroom. "I work with students who have special needs, and I use Repose as a way to help them cultivate self-calming and relaxation skills." In the classroom, she often pairs Repose with soothing music and aromatherapy, which seem to heighten students' receptivity to the experience. "Once they've tried Repose a few times, my students really take to it. They seem to really enjoy it!"

CHAPTER 3

How was Repose Discovered?

Our own discovery of Repose came in an unexpected manner. We had the privilege of living in Italy for three months. During that time, we observed some key differences in the Italian and American lifestyles. Most notably, we were struck by differences in the notion of time. The Italian language has two distinct terms related to time: one is *ora*, which refers to elapsed time and its measurement, and the other is *tempo*, which refers to the pacing or rhythm of life. Relative to Americans, Italians are extremely aware of the importance of pacing, and especially of pauses.

In many Italian towns, shops and businesses close down at midday for a 3-4 hour *pausa*. During that time, people may rest, spend time with friends and family, or enjoy a leisurely meal. Streets empty and entire commercial districts turn into ghost towns. When everything reopens in the late afternoon, people seem reinvigorated. There is none of that "2:30 feeling" which drives Americans to consume energy drinks and other stimulants during the middle of the afternoon.

We returned to the U.S. with the intention of incorporating more pauses into our daily routine. One warm Sunday afternoon, while strolling through a park, we found a spot that seemed particularly inviting. As we lay on the grass under a shady tree, we just fell into the Repose position. Within a few minutes, we both noticed the blissful sensations that were spreading through our bodies. It felt as if we were sails filling with a very uplifting energy. There was something unmistakable about this particular position that seemed to be having the same effect on both of us. After lying in Repose for several minutes, we noticed a qualitative difference in our overall energy levels and well-being. We knew we had found a "potent pause" that could make all the difference not only in our own lives but also in the lives of others.

Life in Repose
Dane, 28, social worker managing programs for at-risk youth

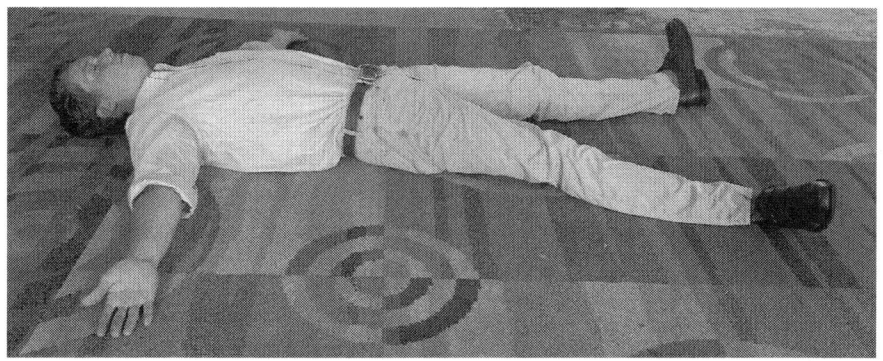

Dane began incorporating Repose into his life at a time when he was experiencing major challenges both at home and in the workplace. The extreme stress he was undergoing manifested itself in a variety of physical symptoms, including shoulder and stomach tension, teeth grinding, and nausea.

Repose helped Dane manage these symptoms. "Although I still felt the stress, five minutes of Repose twice a day offered a break from the symptoms." This relief would last for several hours, until the next Repose break. "Without Repose, it would have been extremely difficult to get through that time and still be able to balance my work and family responsibilities."

For Dane, the benefits of Repose are clear. "Repose makes me feel calm and peaceful." Afterwards, he feels relaxed and invigorated. "My tensions melt away and my mind is clear. I notice this after every Repose session."

His favorite Repose experience was his first. "It was a long day where I sat in a hard wood chair for an extensive period of time. So I was anxious to stretch my legs and get some exercise but I was extremely fatigued from sitting for about nine hours in one place. I felt so listless that I began to give up on the idea of getting in a workout. Additionally, I had been somewhat disappointed with the quality of my training sessions at the gym recently and struggled to drum up enthusiasm.

"I had only learned of Repose earlier that day, and so I decided to give it a shot. When I got on the bed and found a comfortable Repose position, it was as if I was being transported into another dimension. It started almost immediately after I closed my eyes. I lay there experiencing the deep solitude Repose brought me for what seemed like a few minutes but then I glanced at the clock and noticed that much more time had gone by than I would have guessed! It was an incredible experience, only made better by my trip to the gym afterward. I went in and had the best workout I have had in over a year."

Dane would like to see more people try Repose, especially those who think they are too busy to lie down for a few minutes during a hectic workday. "Although it may be difficult to make Repose a priority, I can tell you that after five minutes in Repose I have experienced an invigoration only comparable to a 60-minute massage AND a long night's sleep."

CHAPTER 4

Is it Meditation?

There are two basic forms of meditation: concentrative and mindfulness. Concentrative meditation focuses attention on a specific target such as a sound (*mantra*), visual image (*mandala*), gesture (*mudra*), or physical pose (*asana*). Mindfulness meditation does virtually the opposite, expanding attention to encompass as much as possible without focusing on any one object.

Repose is not like either of these. When you are in Repose, you can direct your attention however you want. You do not need to focus on anything in particular or keep from focusing. In Repose, your mind can do what comes naturally. Unlike meditation, Repose is not a discipline or practice. To experience Repose, you do not need to adhere to any specific philosophy or become proficient in any technique. There is no learning curve and no wrong way to be in Repose.

Meditation and Repose do share certain things in common. Both can improve your sense of well-being, giving rise to personal insights and reducing stress. As with meditation, Repose can help you break free of habitual thoughts, perceptions, emotions, sensations, and behavior. Doing Repose on a regular basis can give you a fresh perspective on things, as if you were looking at the world through a new set of eyes. Both meditation and Repose have the potential to open you up to new experiences and stimulate your innate creativity.

Life in Repose
Renate, 72, grandmother and widow of six years

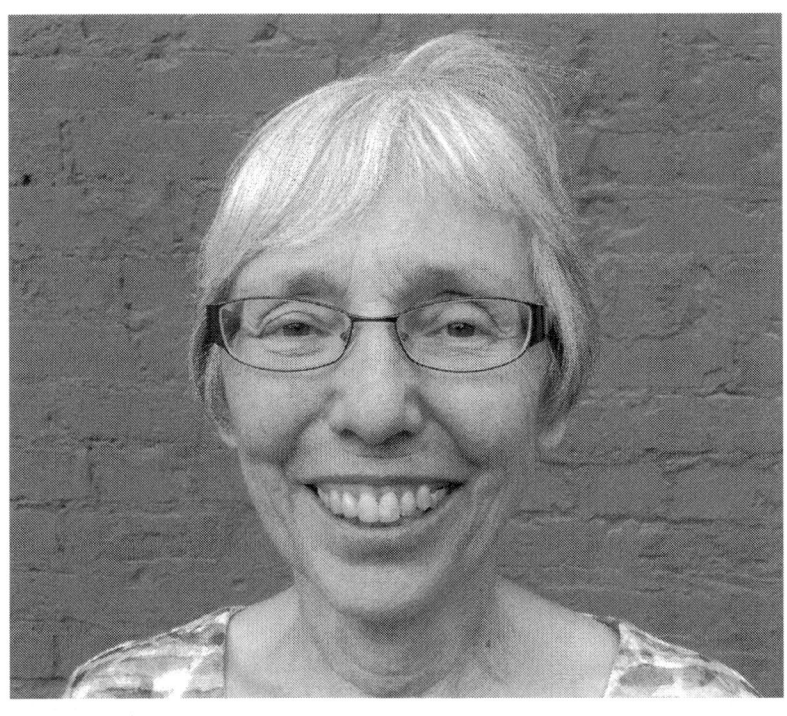

Renate has declared her love of Repose and with good reason. "For six years after my husband died, I had major insomnia, which was frustrating. Then I tried Repose. For the first month, I practiced it religiously three times a day. My sleep pattern began to improve. I was able to fall asleep at night and slept much better. There were at least 15 nights that first month that I didn't take any Valium—for the first time in years—and I slept great. It was amazing!"

What does Renate like best about Repose? "It relaxes and centers me. When I lie in Repose, my body falls into my mattress and feels heavy. Afterwards, I have more energy and feel rejuvenated."

Another quality that draws her is its simplicity. "Repose is so easy and effective. I don't have to do anything."

For a while, Renate assumed that her insomnia was cured, and her Repose breaks became less frequent. Several months passed, and some of her sleep problems returned. "I realized that for me to just practice Repose in the evening when I try to fall asleep or after I wake up at 3 AM is not half as effective as when I practice it religiously three times a day." She also discovered the importance of maintaining a consistent schedule. "I do better when my Repose sessions happen at about the same times every day."

Eventually, Renate returned to her original schedule, which has made a lasting difference in her physical and mental health. "So the moral of the story, which I only fully realize right now, is that I feel much better when I'm doing Repose three times a day."

CHAPTER 5

Is it Relaxation?

Repose bears a resemblance to standard relaxation techniques, especially in terms of the benefits derived from doing it. As with these other techniques, Repose can help to relieve stress and improve overall well-being. But there are two important differences.

Firstly, Repose is much easier to learn and to carry out than most relaxation techniques. In autogenic training, for instance, the practitioner has to repeat a set of visualizations that takes a certain degree of concentration and imagery skill. Biofeedback training involves the use of external devices to monitor physiological functions like heart rate, brain waves, skin conductance and muscle tone. Progressive muscle relaxation (PMR) and self-hypnosis require either extensive practice, the guidance of another individual, or the use of an audio recording. Most breathing and yoga techniques used in relaxation have a learning curve, whereas Repose can be learned in a few seconds and requires no effort whatsoever. There is no cost associated with Repose and no need for either equipment or guidance.

Another important difference is that Repose goes beyond simple relaxation. People who experience Repose on a daily basis report feelings of euphoria, which they describe in a variety of ways: lightness, joy, openness, clarity, energy, and bliss. Some have compared the heightened sense of well-being and connectedness to the experience of a drug "high." But unlike the effects of a psychoactive drug, the enjoyable increase in physical and mental arousal that accompanies Repose can be sustained for extended periods. Whereas tolerance can result from continued drug use, the euphoria produced by Repose does not seem to wear off or diminish over time. Just the opposite can occur. The more time you spend in Repose, the more likely you are to experience its benefits.

Life in Repose
Monyka, 45, mother, teacher, and creative artist

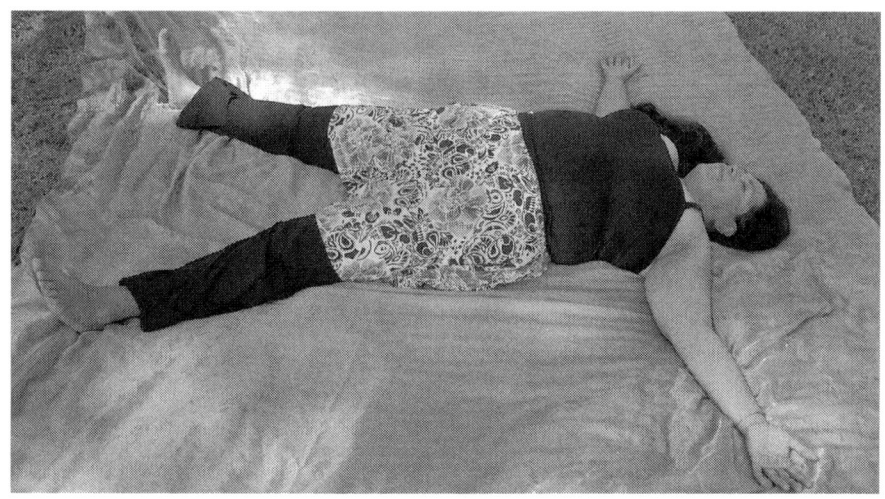

Monyka experiences an immediate sense of peace and balance when she lies down in Repose. "I come to myself, to my center. I observe my thoughts and let them pass. I feel my body stretching, my breath slowing, my brain cooling down, and unwanted thoughts getting released."

Following a Repose session, she feels fresh and able to meet the world anew. "I feel certain that it helps keep me healthy. Repose creates an attitude adjustment, whereby I can choose to be a happy person who knows about self-care. By taking care of myself and maintaining balance in my life, I can be a good role model for my son and my colleagues."

Repose helped Monyka break a habit of choosing caffeine, chocolate, or food for comfort and stress relief at the end of a workday. "When I would come home from school, I used to reach for an unhealthy snack. Now, I lie in Repose instead. I replaced an unhealthy response with a healthy new habit, and it feels wonderful."

Monyka finds Repose especially useful in dealing with acute stress. "I rely on Repose when I'm feeling a headache or an 'oh, no' experience coming on. For me, lying in Repose has become a valuable coping skill." She often recommends Repose, especially to some of her teacher colleagues for their stress-related symptoms. "I know it helps me recuperate from stress, and I am equally confident that it can do the same for others."

CHAPTER 6

What Happens in Repose?

To understand the process by which Repose produces these benefits, let's travel back in time to 1890, when *The Principles of Psychology* by William James first appeared in print. In this work, James introduced ideas about consciousness, will, emotion and a variety of other topics that continue to influence the field of psychology more than a century later.

What makes these ideas so profound is that many of them are counterintuitive. For instance, James proposed that you do not run from a bear because you feel fear but just the opposite. Your body responds rapidly to a dangerous situation such as an encounter with a bear. A signal from your brain to your adrenal glands results in the release of adrenaline and other hormones that trigger an immediate energy surge throughout your body. In an instant, your heart rate and blood pressure increase, pumping nutrients and oxygen to your muscles in preparation to either run from the bear or, as a last resort, try to fend it off. This chain of events is the classic fight-or-flight response that allows your body to use short bursts of energy for a quick escape from danger. The physical arousal associated with fight-or-flight can account for remarkable feats of strength in emergency situations, such as a frail grandmother lifting a two-ton automobile off a child trapped under it.

James proposed that when it comes to emotion, the physical precedes the mental. First, your body becomes aroused and then you feel fear. Your awareness of having an emotion such as fear may be delayed because consciousness is generally slow to emerge. Research in neuroscience has shown that there is a half-second delay between the occurrence of an event and your awareness of it. This delayed reaction means that in a crisis, your body has to kick into gear before you are fully aware of what is going on around you. In terms of your survival, it makes sense that you would start running from the bear before you ever begin to feel fear. If you had to wait to react until you felt the emotion consciously, it would probably be too late. Your awareness of the emotion is almost an after-effect.

James was the first to come up with the notion of *somatic feedback*, which is that the body leads and the mind follows. Once the body produces a set of responses, such as sweaty palms or a racing heart, the mind registers these responses as a specific emotional state. One of the most convincing demonstrations of somatic feedback comes from the study of facial expressions. You can try this demonstration for yourself: Take a (clean) pen or pencil and hold the tip of it in your mouth in one of two ways. First, try holding it with your teeth. Then, hold it only with your lips. You may notice that your facial expression in the first condition more closely resembles a smile and in the second condition is more like a frown. Research participants who are asked to do this task report feeling happier in the first condition than in the second. This shows that the simple act of smiling makes people feel happier, whereas frowning makes them less so.

The idea of somatic feedback can explain a great deal about the benefits of Repose. When asked to describe someone lying in Repose, the two most common adjectives that people choose are: **open** and **receptive**. In fact, every joint in the body is open during Repose. Even the jaw is kept slack. The end result is an open and receptive physical state, which in turn leads to an analogous mental state.

Life in Repose
Tom, 61, community leader interested in yoga, health, ecology, and sustainable economies

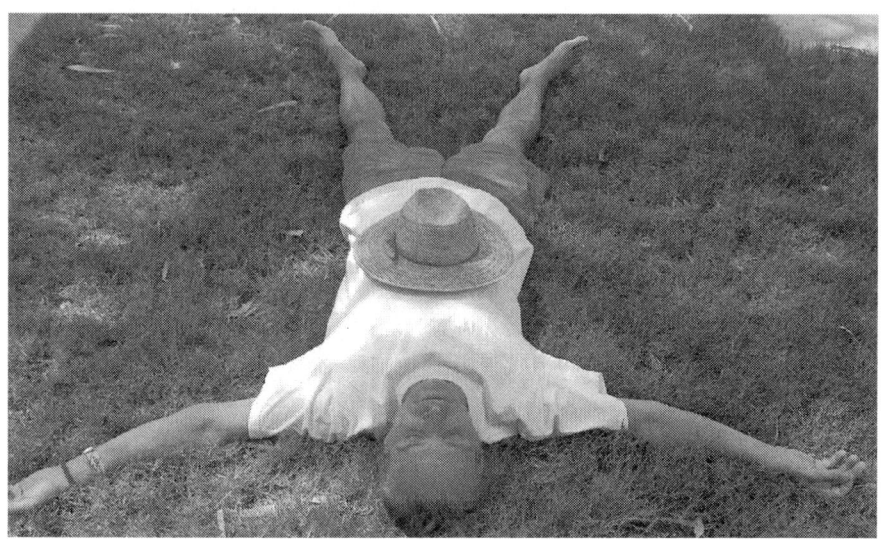

Tom was introduced to Repose when he participated in a research study. After two or three days, he was able to resist distractions and fall into the rhythm of three Repose sessions per day. Then it became a life-changing experience for him.

"Getting the chance to experience Repose at regular intervals during the day promoted a quiet, calm balance for me. It gave me a fresh perspective on the subtle issues recurring in my mind." Tom noticed an enhanced awareness of what was happening inside his body, especially the beating of his heart and the blood flowing in his veins. As the activity of his body settled down, his thoughts become quieter, as well. This created a sensation of physical and mental healing for him.

"After a few minutes of Repose, I felt nourished and refreshed." Months after the study ended, Tom continues to use Repose and sees it as an important life-enhancer. "I believe that Repose can benefit anyone who tries it. Any habit that builds awareness is indisputably valuable, but Repose offers an added bonus of self-healing and relaxation. I have recommended Repose to many people and am happy to spread the word about it."

Tom has noticed that there are times when he almost craves Repose, and he finds those sessions particularly satisfying. "I am driven by the knowledge that Repose opens me up to a healthy, harmonious way of being. It makes me feel lighter, as if a burden were lifted from my mind and body."

Tom also appreciates the fact that Repose is free of charge and so simple to use. He likes taking Repose breaks in the morning, afternoon and evening. "Repose is synced with the rhythms of my day. Three times a day, I get to take a few minutes just for myself. My life can never get too far out of balance when the next Repose break is just around the corner."

He considers Repose to be aptly named. "I enjoy the very idea of being 'in Repose.' That's a great feeling!"

CHAPTER 7

Receptivity and Repose

Researchers who study human consciousness keep stumbling upon the same idea, which is that consciousness can operate in one of two ways.[1] If you are like most people, you spend your waking life in what is known as the *active mode* of consciousness, which is dominated by goals, expectations, and strategies. In this mode, the mind is occupied by a steady stream of thought. The focus of attention moves steadily and rapidly from one thought to the next—often for long periods of time without interruption.

When William James wrote about consciousness in *The Principles of Psychology*, he was basically describing the stream of thought generated in the active mode. Yet James realized that thought alone could not account for all of human experience. "There are two ways of knowing things," he asserted, "knowing them immediately or intuitively, and knowing them conceptually or representatively." You are capable of having a direct experience of life that is free of your intellect. This immediate and intuitive way of knowing is the function of a second mode of consciousness, known as the *receptive mode*.

In the receptive mode, the stream of thought that characterizes the active mode does not seem to exist. This mode relies more on images and sensations than on logical thought. Attention in the receptive mode seeks to draw in everything at once rather than jumping from one thought to the next. The emphasis is on "intake of the environment rather than manipulation," says psychologist Arthur Deikman, who has written extensively about this mode of consciousness. Deikman points out that receptivity should not be mistaken for passivity. "'Letting it' is an activity, but a different activity than 'making it'."[2]

Boundaries seem to get blurred in the receptive mode. Perhaps the most interesting of these is the one that separates "self" from "other." When Deikman asked a group of research participants to stare at a blue vase for 40 half-hour sessions spanning several months, many of them reported the experience of losing themselves in this task. Their sense of identity or separateness seemed to give way to a feeling of connectedness ("I really began to feel, you know, almost as though the blue and I were perhaps merging or that that the vase and I were one"). Psychologists attribute this type of experience to the capacity for *self-transcendence*, which is defined by three characteristics: (1) self-forgetfulness, (2) identification with something or someone beyond the self, and (3) acceptance or openness to spiritual ideas and possibilities.[3]

In essence, self-transcendence is the capacity to connect with something greater than oneself, including humanity, nature, God, or ideals like truth, love, and compassion. Ironically, self-transcendence serves your self-interest. You are most likely to feel good about yourself when you are able to see yourself as more than just an isolated, independent entity and when you can recognize your connection to something bigger. In a recent study, we found a dramatic positive impact of self-transcendence on happiness and overall well-being.[4]

You might think that consciousness can only exist in either the active or receptive mode at any one time, but not in both. This does not seem to be the case, however. There is evidence that the two modes of consciousness can operate at the same time. In fact, the receptive mode appears to be an ongoing backdrop to all of our conscious experience. The reason we may not be aware of it has to do with the intensity of the signal. This intensity can be compared to sound volume. Suppose you had two channels of music playing at the same time. The louder channel is probably going to drown out the softer one. Similarly, the receptive mode may not get noticed if most of your attention is being consumed by the barrage of thoughts generated in the active mode. Although the receptive mode may be in the background, it is still shaping your conscious experience.

So, what does this all have to do with Repose? It seems that Repose works like a "pause" button, giving you a temporary break from the seemingly endless stream of thought coming through the active mode of consciousness. In this pause, the receptive mode emerges from the shadows so that you can immerse yourself fully in it. When this happens, you gain access to an experience that transcends logical thought and even your own sense of self. This experience turns out to have enormous physical and psychological benefits.

Interestingly, the silencing of the active mode and the emergence of the receptive mode happen simply as a result of lying supine with arms and legs extended. Early in his research on the two modes of consciousness, Deikman observed that physical posture can play an important role in inducing one or the other:

> Try thinking about a problem while lying flat on your back, and then...thinking about the same problem while sitting upright. You will notice that maintaining a directed, logical stream of thought is much easier in the upright position. This can be understood as a function of two different states, initiated by postural changes, but not determined by postural changes alone. It is possible to think logically while supine but it is more difficult. Our active-mode activities develop in conjunction with an upright posture, while receptivity originated in the reclining, infant state.[5]

This brings us back to the notion of somatic feedback. Whether or not posture alone is enough to induce a specific state such as receptivity may be subject to debate, but it seems clear that posture can be relied upon to do the heavy lifting in terms of guiding us into these states. Consider, for example, recent research on *high-power poses* such as the one shown here (which has been referred to as the "Wonder Woman" pose):

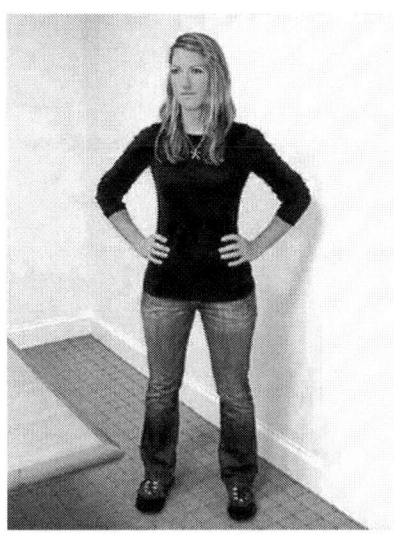

Holding one of these poses for as little as two minutes can raise your testosterone levels by 20%, lower your cortisol levels by 25%, and increase the likelihood that you will be rated by an interviewer as perceptive, confident, enthusiastic, authentic, comfortable, and captivating. In her analysis of these findings, Harvard psychologist Amy Cuddy concludes that "our bodies change our minds."[6]

And this is exactly the case with Repose. The physical receptivity of this position induces psychological receptivity, which in turn triggers what might be called an "upward spiral" of beneficial outcomes. The body does the work in bringing about this chain of events because Repose involves virtually no effort on the part of the mind.

Interestingly, Cuddy's reasoning about why high-power poses are effective also applies to Repose. In high-power poses, she claims, your body is in a more expansive posture than in lower-power poses, in which you might make yourself smaller in various ways, such as hunching over or folding your arms. Repose is the most expansive posture you can assume. When you are in Repose, your body is as open and extended as it can be. If the power of a pose is determined by how large it makes your body feel and appear, then Repose should be viewed as the ultimate high-power pose.

Life in Repose
Martha, 67, acupuncturist and Reiki master

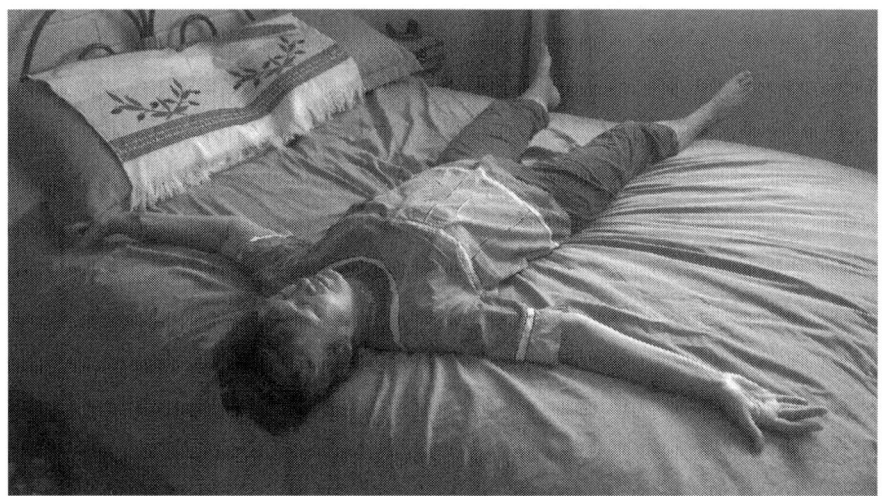

When Martha was first introduced to Repose, she assumed that it was something with which she was already familiar. "I do a lot of yoga, and every session ends with *Shavasana*, also known as 'corpse pose.' In *Shavasana*, we lay face up on the floor with our arms about six inches away from the body, palms up, and our legs lightly splayed. I thought Repose would be a variation on *Shavasana* and expected a similar response on my part: a deep sense of relaxation and well being. But I was in for a surprise!

"With my arms straight out to my sides and my legs wide open as well, I initially felt very exposed. That feeling of vulnerability could be pretty strong, like the time that I practiced Repose on a picnic bench in a city park. But I found that I loved being so open and expanded. I started referring to Repose as 'angel pose.' I would say to myself, 'Okay, honey, it's time to go do angel pose.'"

During the month that she was doing Repose three times a day as part of a research project, Martha caught the flu. "At times, I felt really miserable, but then I would lie in angel pose and it became like an oasis for me." One of the most common experiences Martha would have while in Repose was a feeling of lightness. "I would get this beautiful sensation, as if I could just open up and float away. I got so that I knew exactly when the seven minutes were up, because there would be that delightful 'lifting off' effect right at the end."

Since having the flu, Martha has developed a seizure disorder. "With the seizures, my energy has changed dramatically. I tire relatively easily. But when I feel that way, I use the angel pose to revive myself. Just those few minutes and I feel much better." Martha is grateful to the research project for getting her to use Repose on a daily basis, which she continues to do. "It is one of the tools I can rely on," she concludes. "Whenever I lie down to relax, my body now spontaneously falls into angel pose. Seven minutes later, I'm flying."

CHAPTER 8

Which Thoughts are Most Conducive to Repose?

We often get requests for suggestions about how to occupy one's mind during Repose. The reason we resist such requests is that Repose does not require mental effort. It is neither a mental discipline nor a spiritual practice. Any suggestions we might offer could cause people to mistake Repose for one or the other.

As we have already mentioned, nobody needs to be taught how to be in Repose. It simply comes naturally. In Repose, the body leads and the mind follows. The receptive physical state created during Repose gives rise to an analogous mental state. When this happens, mental activity slows down of its own accord, and a very enjoyable and peaceful state ensues.

Having said this, we have received feedback from individuals who experience Repose on a daily basis, many of whom say they focus on certain types of thoughts to help ease them into the right frame of mind. Here are a few strategies that seem to work for these individuals:

- Focus on a word that corresponds to the experience you desire to have in Repose, such as: "BLISS," "PEACE," "RAPTURE," or "BALANCE."
- Imagine yourself lying in a beautiful, inspiring place on a perfect day.
- "There is nowhere else you need to be and nothing else you need to do. Just be present in this moment."
- Take slow deep breaths. As you breathe in, feel yourself becoming more relaxed. As you breathe out, let go of anything that is causing you strain or tension.
- Keep the following set of intentions in mind: "Here is life. Let it fill me. Let its sweetness flow through me. Let it sweep me away and carry me home. May I come to life. May I be in the flow of life. And may I welcome you to come to life with me."

- As you breathe in, say to yourself, "Fill with love," and as you breathe out, "Radiate joy."

If these or other strategies are helpful, then we encourage using them. But we know from our research as well as our personal experience with Repose that people derive the benefits of Repose without having to adopt a particular strategy or making an effort to clear their minds.

Life in Repose
KC, 72, recovery support specialist

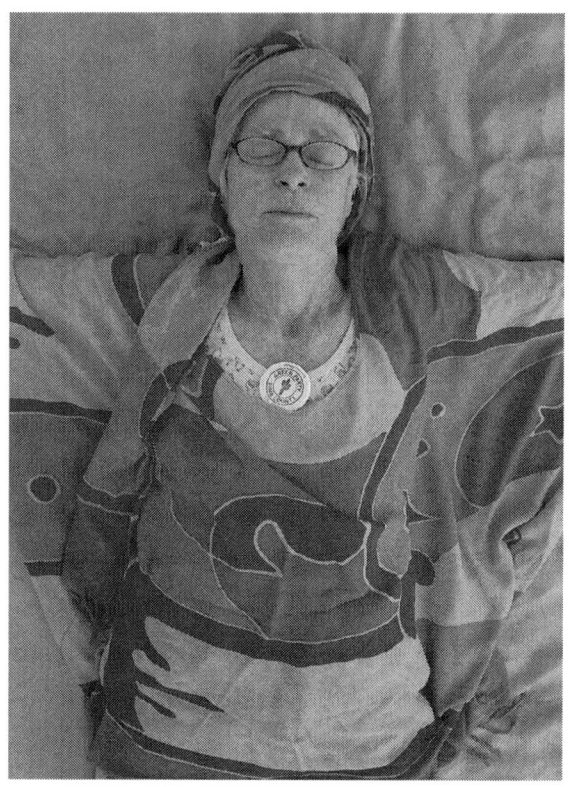

For KC, Repose is an important part of a health regimen that saved her life. "Two years ago, I had Stage 4 liver disease, which is pretty much a death sentence. Today, I have a normal healthy liver. That type of recovery is almost unheard of." Her recovery began with a decision to eliminate stress from her life as much as possible.

"Repose has been great for that. When I lie in Repose, I just 'chill out' and let go of any stress I might be feeling." KC can tell when the benefits of Repose begin taking effect because she feels a strong sense of relief. "It's like getting a daily tune-up. After Repose, I feel like I'm good for another 500 miles."

KC is an energetic person who is always on the go. At first, she had to get used to the idea of stopping everything she was doing in order to take a Repose break. But she quickly discovered how valuable it was to do so. "Learning to take time out for Repose helps with my peace of mind, which for me is a matter of life and death."

For KC, Repose is better when it is shared. "I love lying in Repose with the cat on one side of me and the dog on the other." She also enjoys the experience of Repose in a group setting. "Recently, a musician friend played his didgeridoo while a bunch of us were lying in Repose. It was one of the best feelings you could ever imagine! The sound vibrations just added to the waves of bliss already moving through my body during Repose. Having several of us sharing in the experience just seemed to intensify it that much more."

As a mental health professional, KC considers Repose to be a potentially valuable tool in the treatment of addiction and other mental health issues. "I think that it could help control drug and alcohol cravings. Instead of surrendering to temptation, the person could surrender to Repose." KC also maintains that Repose can be useful for individuals dealing with anxiety or depression. "It's a great way to ride out the storm."

KC feels a strong sense of gratitude for the things that have helped her heal. "I am alive and healthy at a time when I should be long dead. If I hadn't figured out how to get rid of stress, I wouldn't be here right now. Repose has been a really important part of that."

CHAPTER 9

Why is Repose such a "Potent Pause"?

In Repose, the active mode of consciousness takes a brief pause. The word *Repose* itself means "to pause again" in Latin. Every time you are in Repose, your thought processes are silenced for a little while. This mental silence is potent because it provides an opportunity for stress relief, health, improved mental acuity, and happiness.

Stress Relief. Stress is your body's response to a perceived threat. We have already seen that an encounter with a bear triggers a chain reaction in the body that delivers energy to the muscles and mobilizes your body's defenses. In modern urban life, you are unlikely to come across life-or-death situations like a bear attack very often. Yet stress levels seem to be skyrocketing. Why is that?

Your body may react to worries, fears, concerns, and preoccupations as if they were life-or-death situations. If you are consumed with negative thoughts about your job, relationships, home, or finances, your body interprets these problems as a bear attack. Psychological stress produces the same reaction as a physical threat. In terms of how your body reacts, there is no difference.

Repose offers a simple and effective way to alleviate stress. For thousands of years, philosophers have debated the "mind-body problem." With respect to stress, we offer this inversion: **no mind, nobody, no problem**. When you take a break from your thought processes ("no mind") and from yourself ("nobody"), your stress just goes away ("no problem"). Stress is fueled by mental activity. Take a break from that and you lighten your load.

The heaviest load of all is the self. All of your problems are personal. When you think about possible sources of stress in your life, the inner dialogue may sound something like this: *I hate **my** job… This person really annoys **me**…**My** car won't start…I can't afford it…**My** kids are driving **me*** *crazy...She doesn't like **me**...**I** need a vacation.* Your stress begins with issues of "I," "me," and "my." If you had no investment in any outcome, no attachment and no expectations, your problems would dissipate. Just consider what happens when you go to sleep angry, sad, or anxious. Often, those feelings are gone when you wake up. That is because you are able to escape your burdens for a few hours while you sleep. Your waking concerns do not follow you into deep sleep because you essentially stop existing—even for a few moments. When some people are awakened from deep sleep, they are so disoriented that they may not be able to remember where they are or even who they are. In some cases, they report having lost all awareness of themselves. A milder version of this experience has been reported by individuals coming out of Repose. Without a sense of self, stress just disappears.

Improved Health. About 77% of physical health issues are stress-related.[7] Here is a list of common disorders that have been linked to stress:

Acne	Depression	Insulin Resistance
Alcoholism	Dermatitis	Myofascial Pain
Alzheimer's Disease	Diabetes	Obesity
Anxiety	Drug Addiction	Panic Attacks
Arthritis	Fibromyalgia	Phobias
Asthma	Hair Loss	Posttraumatic Stress Disorder
Bipolar Disorder	Heart Disease	Psoriasis
Cancer	Heartburn	Sexual Dysfunction
Chronic Fatigue Syndrome	Herpes	Shingles
Chronic Pain	High Blood Pressure	Sleep Disorders
	Infections	Stroke[8]

The list includes five of the 10 leading causes of death in the U.S: heart disease (#1), cancer (#2), stroke (#4), Alzheimer's disease (#6), and diabetes (#7).[9] In all of these disorders, inflammation plays an important role. Inflammation is the immune system's response to a possible threat. Chemical markers such as cytokines and c-reactive proteins attach themselves to foreign invaders (e.g., bacteria or viruses) or to damaged and dead cells. White blood cells are delivered to the area to destroy and remove the marked cells. Nearby blood vessels become dilated so that they can deliver oxygen and nutrients to the white blood cells.

Although inflammation is needed for the prevention and healing of infectious diseases, there can be too much of a good thing. When the body is out of balance, inflammation tends to make matters worse. Dilated blood vessels can deliver oxygen and nutrients to cancer cells, hastening their growth. Inflammation of blood vessels that already have a buildup of plaque can cause additional irritation and narrowing, which increases the risk of heart disease and stroke. In the brains of Alzheimer's patients, inflammation can accelerate the progress of the disease. The release of cytokines by white blood cells can damage insulin-producing cells in the pancreas, helping to trigger the onset of Type II diabetes.

What causes these problems? One explanation is that we are living in an increasingly toxic world, which is causing our immune systems to work overtime. Inflammation can be triggered by environmental pollutants, certain types of foods, microbes that are becoming increasingly tougher and more drug resistant, and—of course—stress. Chronic psychological stress releases the hormone, cortisol, which normally regulates inflammation and keeps it under control. Cortisol is part of the body's short-term response to stress. When a stressor endures for more than a few hours or days, cortisol continues to get pumped into the blood stream until it overloads the body's capacity to absorb it. Eventually, the immune system becomes insensitive to it, which leads to runaway inflammation.

By interrupting the pattern of thoughts and emotions leading to stress, Repose helps get inflammation under control. In this way, Repose can lower the risk of health problems associated with runaway inflammation.

Mental Acuity. Are you interested in sharpening your mental abilities, such as attention, memory, problem-solving, and creativity? If so, you are not alone. Americans spend over $100 million dollars annually on materials and training programs intended to improve their mental acuity. Unfortunately, these methods have only limited benefits because most mental abilities do not get better simply by trying harder. In fact, effort may be counterproductive in some cases.

Consider what happens when you're trying to recall someone's name. This might be a person whom you've met a few times or even one you know extremely well. You might be able to picture their face but for some reason, you have a mental block when it comes to their name. Maybe you know that it starts with the letter "S," although you can't even be sure of that. You rack your brain looking for clues. You might even try to generate names of people you know: Sharon, Suzie, Sally, Simona.

Unfortunately, none of those are the name you need, and you don't seem to be getting any closer to your answer.

Then, while you're lying in bed or in the shower it just comes to you: *Her name is Stella!* Why was it so hard to come up with that name? Memory researchers would say that you lacked the proper retrieval cues to access it. Remembering something can be like fishing, and the cue is the hook. It takes just the right hook to catch that Stella-fish, if you will. You may need to form some type of mental association, based perhaps on how the name sounds (like "stellar") or on someone else you know by that name (Stanley Kowalski's wife). In this case, the hooks you are using are catching the wrong fish. You can recall other names beginning with an "S" but not Stella. These other names may actually make matters worse, creating interference that prevents you from accessing the name you need.

The much more challenging question is: Why did the name come to you when it did? When you're lying in bed or taking a shower, the active mode of consciousness relaxes and the receptive mode takes over. In this mode, there is no interference from other memories. You have emptied the pond of all fish. When you reintroduce fish back into the pond, you can bring back only the ones you want to catch. Even though the hook you are using has not changed, your chances of catching the right fish with it have increased greatly.

Repose rests the mind in a way that can benefit not just memory but also attention. Consider how hard it is to concentrate when you are feeling stressed. Powerful emotions such as worry, anxiety, and fear can consume your mental energy and keep you from concentrating on the task at hand. It is not surprising that being in a relaxed and receptive state can increase your focus. Taking just a few minutes out of a busy workday to do Repose can have a major impact on productivity by soothing your mind and shutting out distractions.

Repose also has important applications related to problem-solving. For years, researchers have known that working harder on a problem is not necessarily the best way to solve it. Sometimes, you might get stuck in unproductive ways of thinking about a problem, causing you to chase red herrings and dead ends. You may even feel that the harder you try to reach a solution, the more you end up going around in circles. When the old ways of thinking are simply not working, one of the most effective things you can do is to shut things down. There is a reason we say "Let me sleep on it." A few hours of sleep can give your active mode of consciousness a break, after which you are able to approach the same problem with an entirely new perspective. But you may not need an entire night's sleep to achieve this effect. A brief session of Repose can serve as a RESET button, clearing out the cobwebs and giving you a fresh take on the problem at hand.

It would make sense, then, that Repose would have a similar effect on creativity. One of the great mistakes that psychology has made is to equate creativity with thinking. The reports of visionaries and pioneers in almost every field suggest that something else is taking place during the creative process. These individuals often describe a receptive state in which ideas and images come effortlessly. Various means have been used to induce this state. For instance, Carl Jung would go to his lakefront property and stare out at Lake Zurich for several days before starting on a new writing project. A biographer of the Beatles observed that when John Lennon and Paul McCartney wrote songs together, "each seemed to be in a trance" as they sat playing their respective instruments for hours at a time.[10]

Receptivity appears to be the key to creative insight. In *The Courage to Create*, Rollo May wrote, "The receptivity of the artist must never be confused with passivity. Receptivity is the artists' holding himself or herself alive and open…Such receptivity requires a nimbleness, a fine-honed sensitivity in order to let one's self be the vehicle of whatever vision may emerge."[11] Receptivity is heightened when the active mode of consciousness is silenced, as it is during Repose. In the stillness of the receptive mode, you create an opening for something new to arise. Repose is particularly conducive to creative expression because of how it lets you tap into the receptive mode unencumbered by the mental activity of your intellect.

Happiness. One of the most compelling reasons to do Repose is the happiness you will derive from it. Many people who try Repose report having experiences of bliss while doing it. And there seems to be a carryover effect from doing Repose regularly. The positive feelings that are elicited by Repose can often be sustained throughout the day.

This is not surprising. The human mind is the ultimate source of all unhappiness. Certain thoughts and emotions can have a negative impact on your psychological well-being. You might get consumed by thoughts that trigger feelings of anger, depression, anxiety, jealousy, or hatred. And you may be all-too-familiar with the experience of rumination, when you keep replaying the same thoughts obsessively. Over and over again, you might relive painful memories and revisit your most intractable problems—even to the point of disrupting your sleep, elevating your stress levels, and denying yourself simple enjoyment or peace of mind.

In Repose, you give your mind a rest. By interrupting the barrage of thoughts and emotions generated in the active mode, you are able to liberate yourself from the source of all unhappiness. As we saw earlier, the image of someone in Repose conveys the sense of being carefree. This image is consistent with the actual experience. In Repose, you can let go of all your worries and concerns. Most importantly, you can take a break from yourself. When you get past your limited sense of self, you connect to something much greater. Research has shown that this experience of self-transcendence is not only a predictor of happiness but also a cause of it.[12]

Although most people realize they have the ability to make themselves miserable through their thought processes, they have a harder time believing that happiness is within their control. Our society views happiness as a function of circumstance. The very origin of the word is from the Icelandic *happ*, meaning fortune or luck. Implied is the idea that happiness is determined by variables that are unpredictable and outside of one's control. Perhaps this is because people seem to be happiest when they lose themselves in the moment and essentially disappear. At some level, they may realize that to be happy, they need to get out of their own way. Losing self-awareness, even for a few moments, can be a tremendously powerful experience. This transcendent experience goes by many names: bliss, ecstasy, joy, rapture.

Ironically, the decision to surrender to such experience is completely intentional. In other words, you have some control over your decision to give up control. Repose makes that decision particularly easy. You simply choose to take a few minutes out of your day to lie in Repose. This does not guarantee a transcendent experience. Some people feel restlessness, agitation, or boredom the first time they try Repose. Of course, this is not surprising. If someone is accustomed to the constant chatter of an active mind, they may resist any attempt to silence it—even for a few moments. It may not matter that this activity might be detrimental to their health and productivity. They will still choose an experience that is familiar and unpleasant over one that is unfamiliar ("Better the devil you know than the devil you don't").

Although active minds may put up a fight temporarily, the beauty of Repose is that this resistance stops for most people in a matter of minutes. It is simply the nature of somatic feedback that the physical receptivity of Repose leads to mental receptivity eventually. We have observed that this shift tends to happen in 3-5 minutes for most people who experience Repose on a daily basis. The reason we recommend that Repose sessions last seven minutes is to give ample time for the shift to occur and for the individual to savor it.

Once this shift happens, the mood elevation produced by Repose can last for hours. The key to sustaining this blissful state is to recharge it every few hours with another Repose session. We recommend that Repose be done three times a day, preferably at 9am, 3pm, and 9pm (although this can be modified to fit your schedule). If you spread out your Repose sessions in this way, you will never go more than six hours between sessions during your waking day. The benefits you derive from Repose can be sustained indefinitely, which means that you can remain in a peaceful and balanced state regardless of what is happening around you.

CHAPTER 10

Where's the Proof?

Even though our research program on Repose is only in its inception, we already have strong evidence pointing to the benefits of Repose. For instance, a study we completed in April 2014 showed that Repose can have a dramatic positive impact on physical and mental health.[13]

In the first phase of our study, we assigned 48 participants to one of two groups. The experimental group added three Repose sessions to their daily routine for 30 days, whereas the control group did not. Both groups were tested at the beginning and end of the 30-day period to assess three aspects of their overall health: (1) psychological well-being, which includes happiness, optimism, self-image, social support, and resilience; (2) flourishing, defined as high levels of positivity, psychological functioning, and social functioning ; and (3) physical health, measured by the ability to perform normal daily activities like carrying groceries, bathing or dressing oneself, climbing stairs, bending, and walking. Relative to the control group, the experimental group showed significant improvements in all three areas.

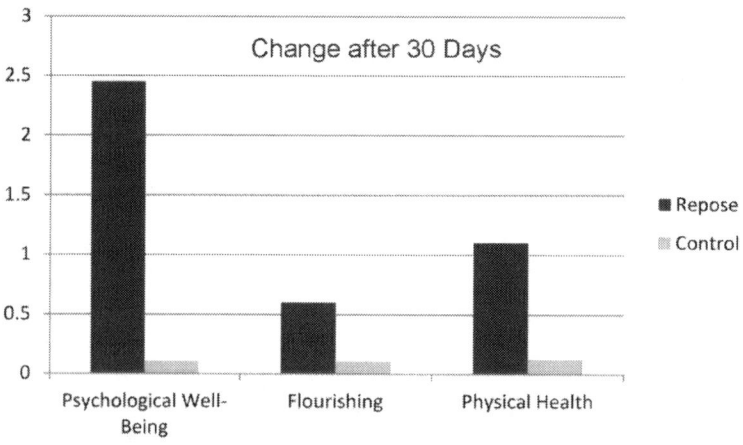

In the second phase of our study, we gave the control group a chance to try Repose for 30 days. They made gains in their overall health and well-being virtually identical to the ones we had observed in our experimental group a month earlier, confirming that the pattern of results obtained in the first phase was not due to chance. Based on these findings, it appears that Repose may have important applications for improving individuals' mental and physical state.

A set of pilot studies conducted by psychology students at the University of Arizona looked at other potential applications of Repose. Here is what these students found:

Stress Reduction. In three different designs, students showed that Repose lowers stress. Looking at her own stress levels, Erica Vega saw a 33 percent drop in those levels after two weeks of Repose.[14]

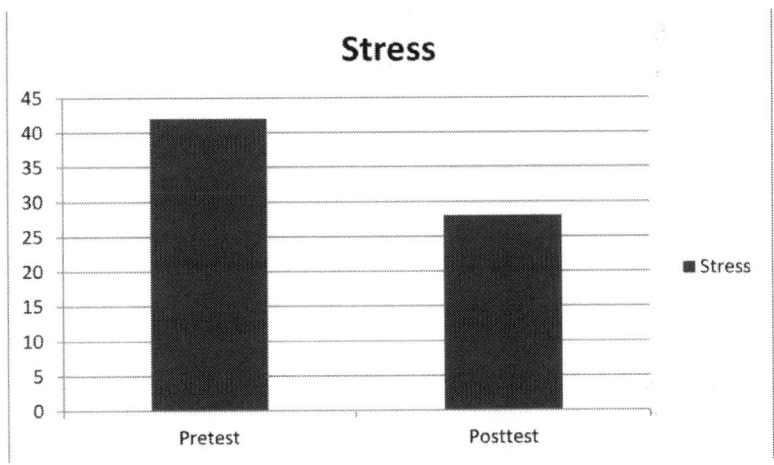

Rebecca Ethington saw a 50 percent drop in her stress levels over a seven-day period, with a steady rate of decline each day.[15] She also observed improvements in the quality and number of hours she was able to sleep each night, which is especially noteworthy given that she conducted this study at a particularly stressful point in the semester, just two weeks before finals.

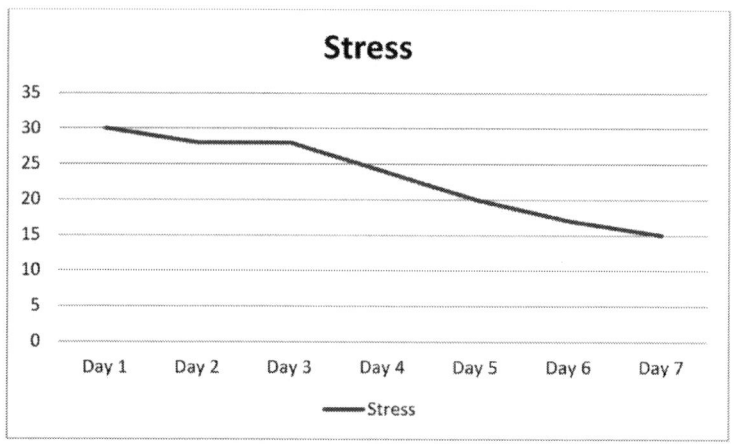

Leigha Galbraith compared the stress levels of two groups: an experimental group that practiced Repose daily for five days and a control group that did not.[16] Stress levels stayed constant for the control group but dropped by 37 percent for the Repose group.

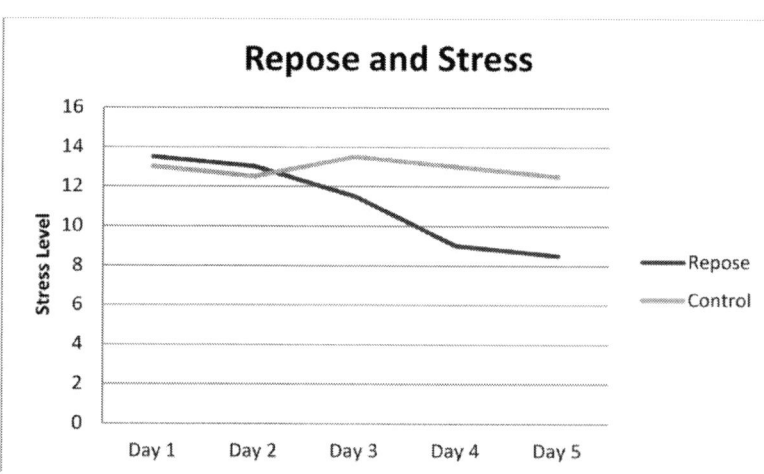

Mental Acuity. Preston Pierce looked at the effect of Repose on mindfulness, which is awareness of what is happening in the present, both internally and in one's surroundings.[17] His mindfulness level improved steadily over an 11-day period in which he practiced Repose daily:

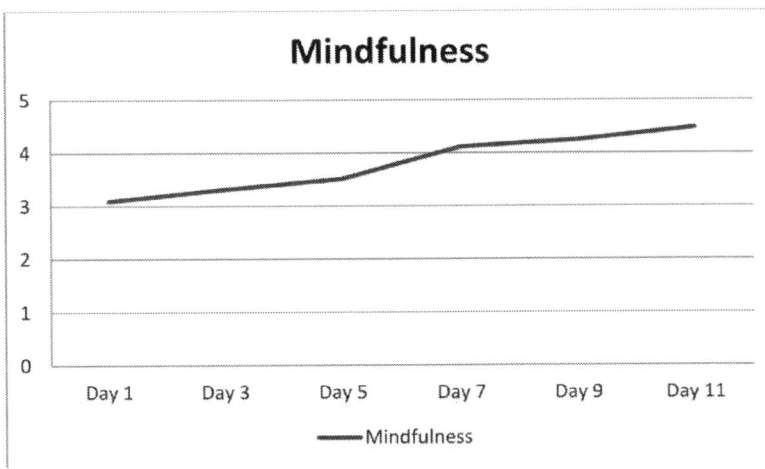

In a pretest-posttest design, Erica Vega found that doing Repose for two weeks improved her accuracy on a test of attention[18] and her productivity as measured by a test of typing speed.

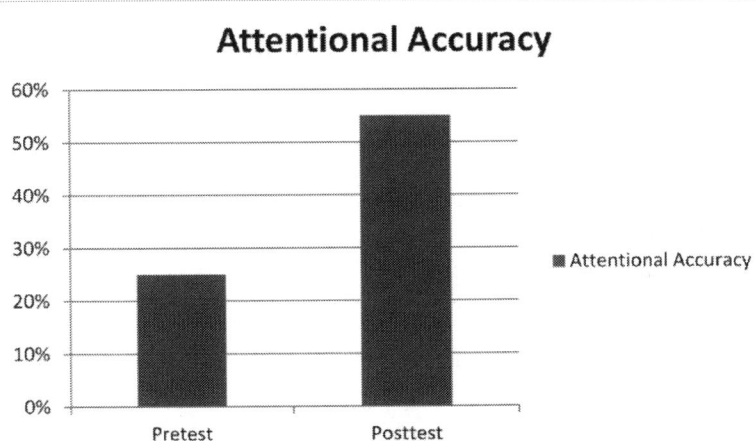

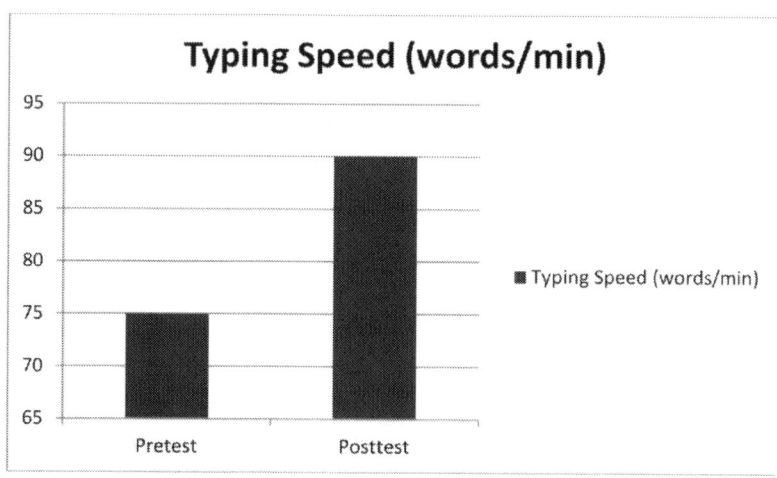

Alyssa Gorce's memory performance was enhanced by Repose.[19] Over a period of three days, she tested her memory for two lists of nonsense syllables (e.g., *wuh, doj, zel*), one of which she studied after seven minutes of Repose and the other after seven minutes of reading a textbook. Her recall in the Repose condition was consistently better than in the control condition:

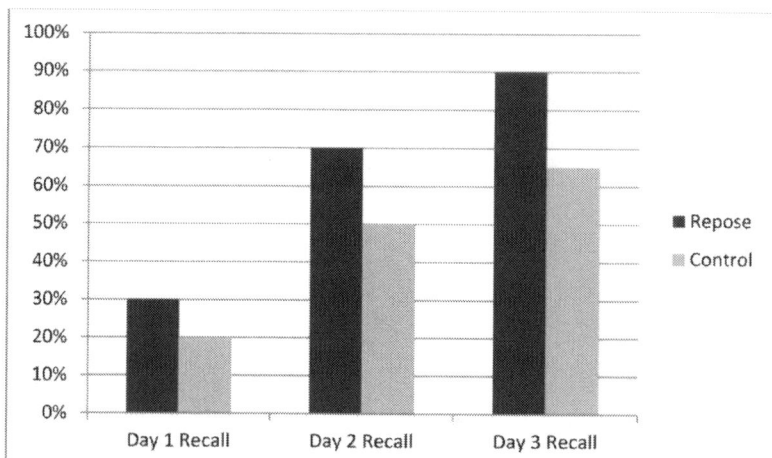

Using the Shapes and Colors Test, Ben Silverman observed that his visual memory was better after seven minutes of Repose than after seven minutes of reading the news online:

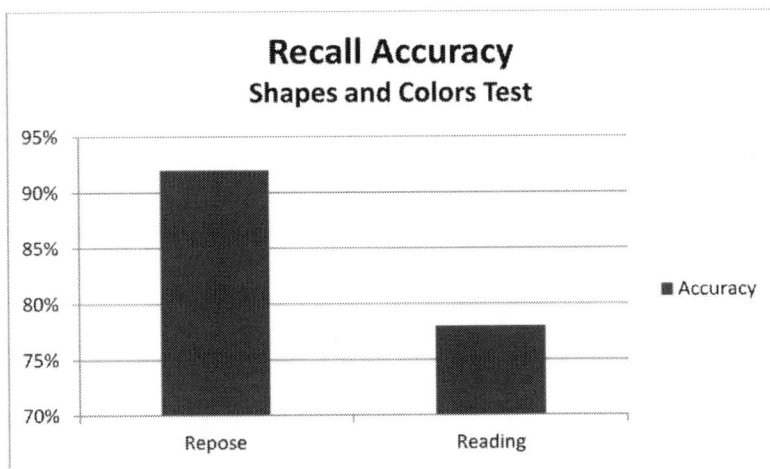

For one student, Repose had a dramatic effect on problem-solving. Laker Dohan looked at incubation effects, which are improvements in one's ability to solve a problem after taking time away from it. He discovered that he could solve more word problems after a five-minute Repose break than he could after reading a textbook for the same amount of time:

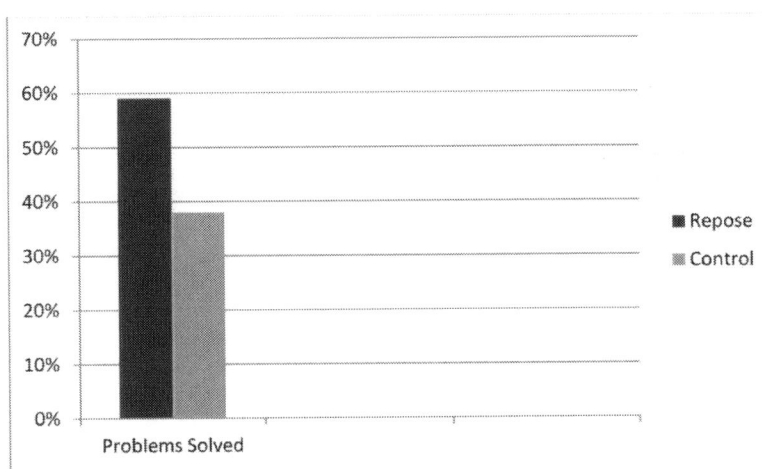

Happiness. Testing herself daily over a two-week period, Kendra Wade[20] observed that she had increased positivity, decreased negativity, and higher ratios of positivity-to-negativity on days when she practiced Repose than on days when she did not:

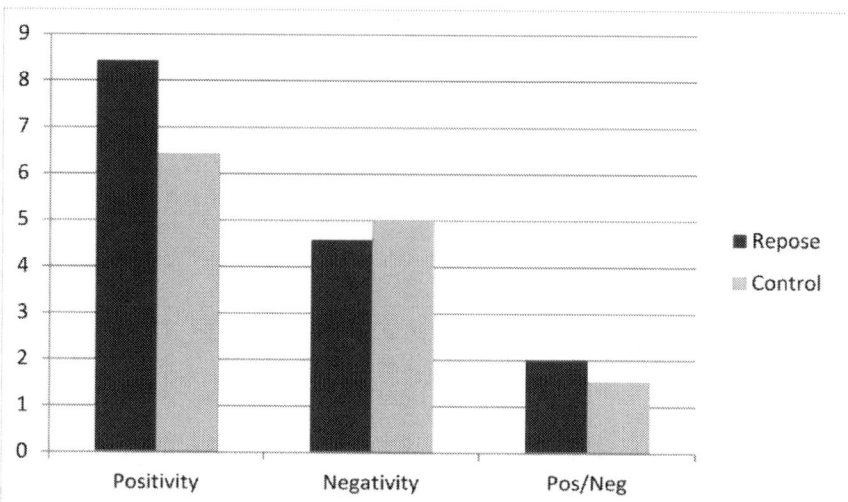

These pilot studies involved very few participants (only one in most cases) and short durations (two weeks or less). Although we are cautious to draw any broad conclusions from them, the fact that they yielded significant effects is extremely promising. Their findings point to several potentially important applications of Repose that we intend to investigate over the next several years.

CHAPTER 11

Where Do We Go from Here?

We expect that you will be hearing much more about Repose in the days ahead. The fact that Repose is effective, free, and simple to use will make it irresistible to researchers, health care providers, and the general public alike. We are about to discover a great deal more about the power of Repose in alleviating stress, improving health, and increasing productivity.

In our own research, we intend to look at the effects of Repose on physical markers of stress, such as c-reactive protein and cortisol. We are in negotiations to start clinical trials of Repose with patient populations suffering from depression, anxiety, and drug and alcohol dependence. We are also interested in testing Repose as a treatment for post-traumatic stress disorder (PTSD), especially given the shortcomings of the government's ongoing multibillion dollar program to treat PTSD in veterans.[21]

The possible applications of Repose seem virtually limitless. We envision a time in the not-too-distant future when the benefits of Repose will be widely recognized. Health spas and clubs will recommend it as an important component of daily health and fitness programs. Because of its effectiveness in alleviating stress, Repose will make its way into hospitals, urgent care centers, and the offices of health care practitioners such as physicians, psychologists, and physical therapists. Drug and alcohol treatment programs will use Repose to help patients manage cravings and to speed up recovery. In schools and workplaces, Repose breaks will serve to refresh and revitalize. Corporate America will see Repose as a simple and effective way to enhance productivity. In conflict mediation sessions, Repose will help to ease tensions and open participants' minds to new possibilities. At festivals, street fairs and other celebrations, thousands of people will come together to share in Repose. Schools, churches, and social clubs will provide the opportunity for Repose at their events. And television networks will schedule daily Repose programming at 9am, 3pm, and 9pm so that millions of viewers can experience Repose together.

We also envision a world in Repose. When hundreds of millions of people around the world start incorporating Repose into their daily lives, the ramifications may be far reaching. Entire societies will be reshaped. People who know what it is to be in Repose will be less drawn to violence, greed, and selfishness. As their feelings of connectedness to others increases, they will demand more compassion and justice from their governments. Businesses that engage in unfair or unhealthy practices will fall away as people stop supporting them. War, exploitation and genocide will not be tolerated. A heightened concern for the welfare of other species and future generations will lead to more sustainable ways of living and stronger environmental policies. Religious conflicts will vanish as people become more aligned with basic spiritual values like loving kindness that cut across all religious differences. Families and communities will thrive as the needs of children, older adults, the sick and the disabled became higher priorities.

Do you doubt that something as simple as Repose could have that kind of an impact? If so, then try it for yourself. For one month, set aside seven minutes for Repose three times a day. Then just observe how it affects your attitudes, health, energy levels, productivity, interactions, and overall well-being. If you have feedback for us, please visit our website, **Repose4all.com**. Your comments, suggestions, and questions are more than welcome. This site includes opportunities to share ideas and stories, get updates on the latest research, track the growing interest in Repose, find out about upcoming events, interact with guest presenters, and more.

Although these resources are invaluable, the best way to understand Repose is through direct experience. Nobody can tell you what it's like to be in Repose or what benefits you will derive from it. That is for you to discover.

Life in Repose
Victor, age 55. Psychologist, author, musician

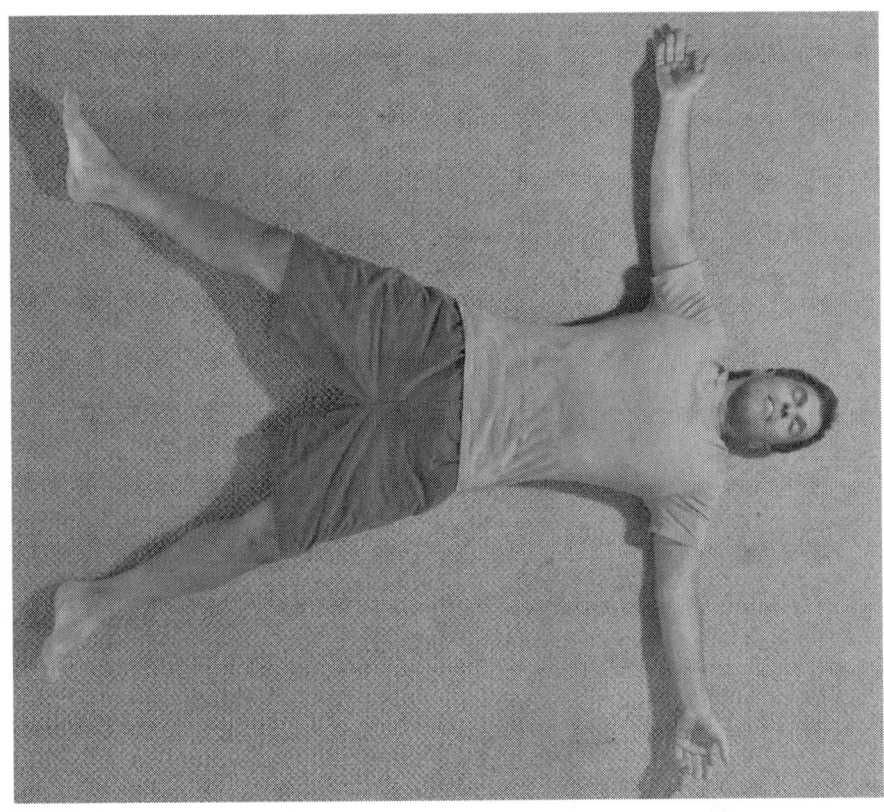

For Victor, Repose was something he had experienced in childhood, although he had no name for it at the time. "I just did it because it felt good. My best friend and I would lie in that position on lazy summer days and just stare at the clouds. This could last for hours, and we never seemed to get tired of it."

When he rediscovered this position as an adult, Victor wondered why it had taken so long to come back to something he had enjoyed so much in his youth. "As soon as I fell into Repose, I could sense the energy flowing freely through my body in ways that it normally doesn't do. That felt incredibly good."

Victor reports an unmistakable transformation that happens within the first few minutes of lying in Repose. "My mind shifts into neutral. I am not struggling or striving for anything." Victor says that his concerns and preoccupations seem to dissipate, and it feels like the tension has been wrung out of his body. "I have moments when I am not even aware of myself as a separate entity in the world. It's total freedom, and it makes me feel energized and relaxed at the same time."

One of the most immediate benefits Victor gained from Repose was that he started losing weight he had gained during a three-month stay in Italy. "Within a couple of months, I also noticed improvement in how my joints felt. For years, I have had pain in my joints—especially my left knee. Now, I rarely experience even the slightest discomfort in my knee or in any other joints."

His creativity and focus also improved. "I have had an explosion of creative output since Repose came into my life, finishing a book, establishing an exciting new direction in my research career, starting a band and composing more music than I had in years." Perhaps most importantly, he feels that he has gained a greater sense of equanimity than ever before. "I know that Repose isn't just something I experience while lying on my back. There is a carryover that affects every aspect of my life. The challenges and drama of life do not seem to faze me. No matter what happens, I know that I am in Repose."

CHAPTER 12

Adaptations and Modifications

You may have physical, emotional, or logistical issues that you feel might prevent you from lying in Repose. Here, we offer a few suggestions that are likely to help.

If getting down on the floor or getting back up is beyond your physical capacity, you may choose to experience Repose from the comfort of your own bed. Repose in bed could be a great way to start or end your day, and you may find that it will help you relax yourself to sleep.

We have no reason to think that Repose is any less effective on a bed than on any other surface. But if you have physical limitations and still wish to experience Repose on the floor, you might want to try an adaptive technique to help you. For instance, you can use a chair to assist you in getting down on the floor. Just follow the three steps shown here

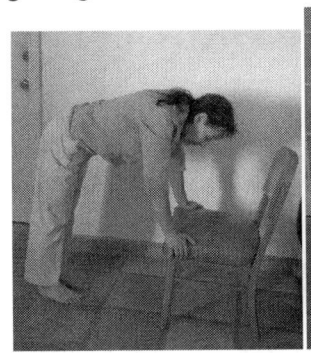 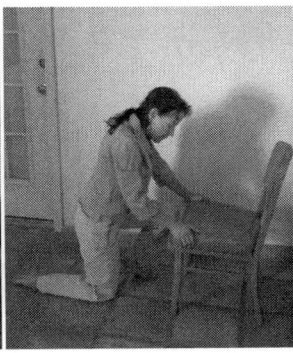 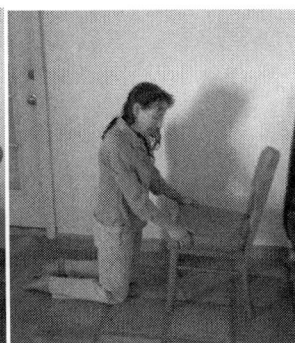

To return to a standing position after Repose, simply reverse these steps.

You may have neck or back pain that gets triggered when you lie flat. In this case, you may want to use props to support your neck, lower back, or knees. Leaving your knees bent while settling into Repose may alleviate some of the pain. Doing a few minutes of deep breathing prior to Repose may be helpful, as well. Another alternative, if you have access to a swimming pool, is to try Repose while floating in the water. You may find it helpful to use a flotation device such as a Styrofoam "noodle." In the water, you should feel no pressure on any part of your back.

You may not need to go to such lengths to be in Repose, however. Being all-too-familiar with lower back pain, we have found that our pain dissipates after a few minutes of Repose on a firm surface. This is purely a personal observation that has yet to be tested in a clinical setting. If you want to find out for yourself, please do so as gently as you can, without causing yourself any additional pain or injury.

If you have pain or restricted range-of-motion in your shoulders, arms, knees, elbows or hips, you might want to place cushions or pillows under those areas. In Repose, the objective is to open up your joints as much as you can **without causing pain or discomfort**. We cannot stress enough the importance of listening to your body and respecting your limits.

Some people have described feelings of vulnerability while lying in Repose. If you have such feelings and they make you uncomfortable, try covering yourself with a sheet or blanket first. You may also want to choose to experience Repose in the most private setting possible. A dark room or a locked door may increase your comfort level significantly.

In terms of comfort, we suggest removing eyeglasses and footwear before entering into Repose. We also prefer loose clothing that doesn't bind or constrict, although you can experience Repose in formal attire or work clothes and still derive all the benefits. In a cold setting, you may want to cover yourself or put on more clothing. In a warm setting, you may need to adjust the temperature, remove items of clothing, or seek shade.

When traveling long distances by car, think about keeping a blanket or mat handy. This allows you to take advantage of unexpected opportunities for Repose. On road trips, we have experienced Repose in parks, rest areas, lawns, beaches, and even on top of our vehicle. As long as you have room to spread out, you can take Repose virtually anywhere.

At work, you may be challenged to find a suitable time and place for Repose. We recommend trying Repose during a lunch or coffee break. You will find that it energizes you and gives you a fresh perspective on whatever you are doing. If you do not have access to an appropriate space (e.g., office or break room) or if you have any concerns about how your co-workers and supervisors will react, save your Repose time for when you get home. Eventually, more workplaces will become receptive to Repose as employers discover the potential benefits, including enhanced productivity and reduced stress.

We have received a number of suggestions for different adaptations, including Repose on a hammock, trampoline, or exercise ball (with knees bent legs at a 90-degree angle and the ball leaning against a wall for stability), although we have not tested the effectiveness of these variations. Individuals with attention deficit or other cognitive issues may benefit from the use of background music or aromatherapy to help relax the mind. It may also be helpful to start with shorter Repose sessions (e.g., one or two minutes), gradually increasing the length of the sessions with increased familiarity and practice.

Feel free to adapt Repose to your specific needs. If you feel more comfortable in a group setting, find willing partners to join you in Repose. We have seen groups of people arrange their bodies into unique formations such as the one shown here:

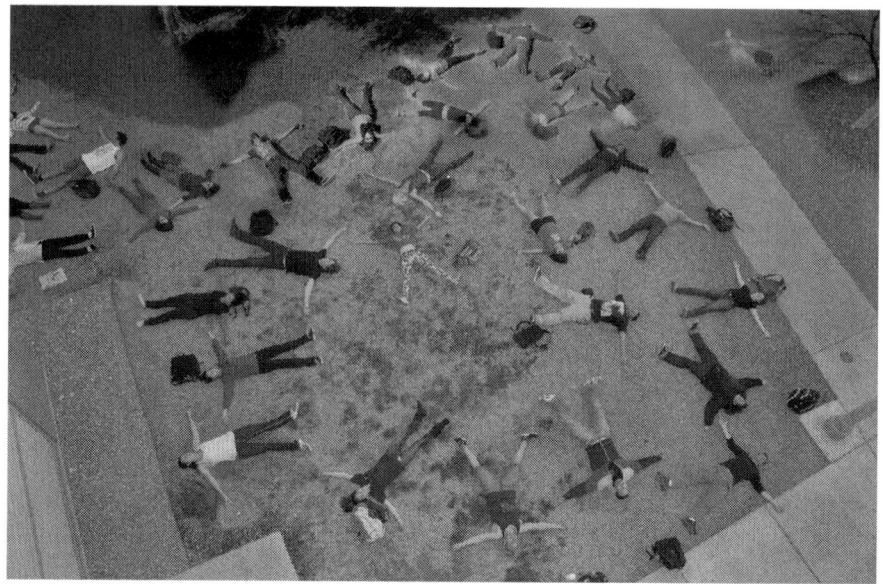

If you and your Repose partners feel comfortable with it, you might try overlapping arms or legs. We have seen small children lie on top of a parent or other adult when families share in Repose. The important thing, of course, is to always respect your partners' boundaries and their need for personal space.

We have even heard from people who claim that merely envisioning themselves in Repose without actually assuming the position is enough for them to receive the benefits of the experience. Like other variations, this "virtual" Repose would need to be tested in order to confirm its effectiveness.

Repose is revolutionary in its simplicity. Although we have discussed a number of variations, the basic idea is always the same: (1) assume an open position with arms and legs extended; (2) hold that position for seven minutes three times daily; and (3) enjoy the physical and psychological benefits. We have experienced such enormous benefits from Repose personally that we have decided to devote our lives to sharing this precious resource with others. Now, it's your turn to reap the rewards that Repose has to offer. Regardless of what happens in your life, may you always be in Repose.

Life in Repose
Jhan, 55, rehabilitation specialist, yoga teacher, and Earth steward

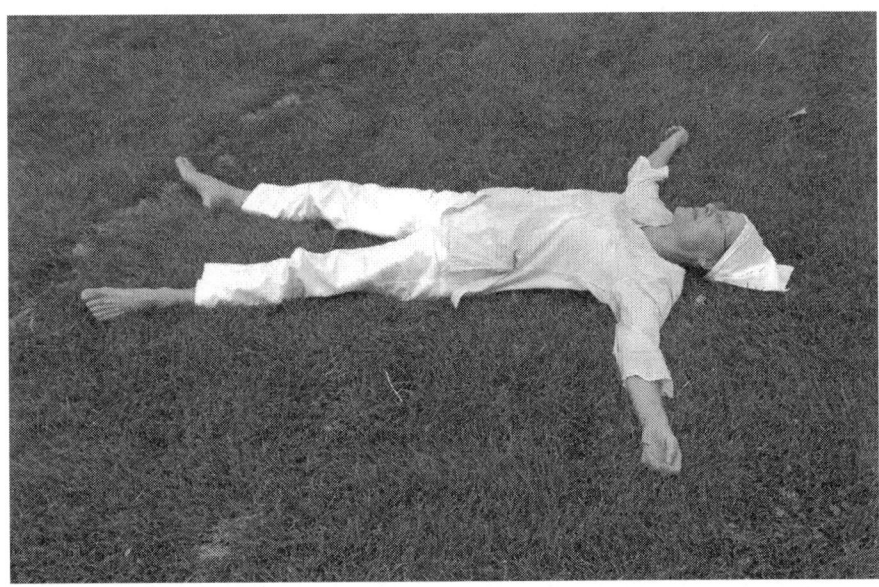

For the past year, Jhan has done Repose anywhere from two to seven times a day. She enjoys the sense of symmetry and balance she experiences in her body during Repose, as well as the opportunity to quiet her thoughts. "Repose gives me 'down time' to go within, which inspires some great intuitive insights and ideas."

Along with her co-author, Jhan shared in the discovery of Repose. "The night before, we had attended a Native American sweat lodge ceremony. The man leading that ceremony voiced a prayer for us to find a new direction in our lives. His prayer was answered less than 24 hours later, when Repose seemed to fall out of the sky and into our laps. Immediately, we recognized it as a life-changing gift to the world—so necessary in these challenging times that require each of us to find peace and equanimity within ourselves.

"Once it was discovered, I quickly christened it *Repose*, because I could see that it gives easy access to a 're-poised' state of bliss, if you will. For me, Repose offers a simple way to immerse myself in the flow of life, much like I imagine it might feel to catch and ride a wave. I also find that it helps me walk away from any snags or obstacles to my innate peaceful state.

Jhan describes her typical Repose experience like this: "When I am in Repose, I feel peaceful, light, and free; expansive, yet intimately grounded into the Earth. For me, Repose creates a sense of being connected to something infinite and mysterious, which I call *lovelight*. The only way I can describe it is as a quality that flows through and encompasses everything and everyone. "

After a few minutes of Repose, Jhan feels rejuvenated, "like I've been washed over, cleansed, renewed, and invigorated." Even on days that are particularly demanding or stressful, Repose has a way of creating a sense of calm and harmony inside of her. "It is as if I am getting recalibrated so that I can return to my natural rhythm and flow. Repose soothes my soul, enhances my awareness of the world around me, and gives me a sense of control over my attitudes and actions."

Notes

1. Shamas, V. A., and Bowers, P. G. (1992). "Hypnosis and Creativity," in E. Fromm and M. R. Nash, eds., *Contemporary Hypnosis Research* (New York, NY: The Guilford Press), 334-363.
2. Deikman, A. J. (1971). "Bimodal Consciousness." *Archives of General Psychiatry*, **25**, 481-489.
3. Cloninger, C. R., Svrakic, D. M., and Przybeck, T. R. (1993). "A Psychobiological Model of Temperament and Character." *Archives of General Psychiatry*, **50**, 975-990.
4. Shamas, V. A., and Garcia, R. A. (Submitted). "Self-Transcendence and Subjective Well-Being: Correlation and Causation."
5. Deikman, A. J. (1973). "Bimodal Consciousness," in R. E. Ornstein, ed., *The Nature of Human Consciousness* (New York, NY: The Viking Press), 67-86.
6. http://www.ted.com/speakers/amy_cuddy
7. http://www.apa.org/news/press/releases/2007/10/stress.aspx
8. http://www.medicinenet.com/stress/related-conditions/index.htm
9. http://www.cdc.gov/nchs/fastats/leading-causes-of-death.htm
10. Hertsgaard, M. (1995). *A Day in the Life: The Music and Artistry of the Beatles*. (New York, NY: Delta Trade Paperbacks).
11. May, R. (1994). *The Courage to Create* (New York, NY: W. W. Norton and Company).
12. Shamas, V. A., and Garcia, R. A. (Submitted). "Self-Transcendence and Subjective Well-Being: Correlation and Causation."
13. Shamas, V. A. and Garcia, R. A. (In Preparation). "The Benefits of Repose."
14. http://prezi.com/w4kqa46zmrro/operation-repose/
15. http://prezi.com/avygzkpfenpq/?utm_campaign=share&utm_medium=copy
16. http://www.prezi.com/vbo2ra_atkmo/repose-stress-reduction/
17. http://prezi.com/ue3xt-kpitqb/?utm_campaign=share&utm_medium=copy

18. http://prezi.com/w4kqa46zmrro/operation-repose/
19. http://prezi.com/qermue7tagm0/relaxation-and-memory/
20. http://prezi.com/ghdkdwvuf8fk/?utm_campaign=share&utm_medium=copy&rc=ex0share
21. http://www.nextgov.com/defense/2014/06/iom-report-defenseva-have-no-clue-if-93-billion-worth-ptsd-treatment-works/86929/

Made in the USA
San Bernardino, CA
14 April 2016